Arteries Cleaned Out Naturally:

Scientific Facts And Fancies

By - Frank W. Cawood
     Rita Warmack
     Janice McCall Failes
     Gayle R. Cawood

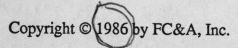
FC&A Publishing
103 Clover Green
Peachtree City, Georgia 30269

Second Edition. Printed and bound by the Banta Company. Cover design by Kip Marshall.

ISBN 0-915099-06-3

Acknowledgements

Many individuals gave of their time and energy in the preparation of this book. We would like to extend a special word of appreciation to:

— Linda Sciullo, for your conscientious typing and proofreading and for your patiently adding our last minute changes.

— Marcia Ulery, for your proofreading and generous assistance with typesetting procedures.

— Mickey Gore, for your long-suffering diligence in rearranging the press date.

— All the supportive staff of FC&A, for your willingness to help.

— But most of all, our thanks and praise is to our Lord and Saviour, Jesus Christ, Who is our very present help in time of need.

... For we are the temple of the living God; as God has said,

> "I will live in them and move among them,
> and I will be their God,
> and they shall be my people ...

SINCE WE have these promises, beloved, let us cleanse ourselves from every defilement of body and spirit, and make holiness perfect in the fear of God.

— II Corinthians 6:16b,7:1
(Revised Standard Version)

Who can ever say, "I have cleansed my heart; I am sinless"?

— Proverbs 20:9
(The Living Bible)

Table of Contents

Introduction

We, the authors of this book, are not medical doctors. We are simply concerned citizens who study scientific research and strive to separate fact from fiction. This book is the prayerful result of much hard work to discover the truth about the prevention and relief of artery disease, especially coronary artery disease which causes half a million deaths annually in the U.S.A., mainly by heart attack. We have investigated and explained the latest methods of medical treatment and management of coronary artery disease and the natural methods of prevention which are accepted by most authorities in the field. We have also examined and described new methods of preventing or relieving coronary artery disease. Some of these new methods of prevention eventually may be "proven" to be effective, while others may be found not to be. In the meantime, they should be tried only under a doctor's care. Use common sense and don't neglect proven methods of prevention and treatment.

This book also reports the new discovery of how the body cleans its own arteries naturally. This exciting, new discovery means that artery disease isn't inevitable. There are many things we can do to help the body keep its arteries clear.

Heart attacks don't have to happen. Most people can avoid them. They are not an inescapable fact of aging. As a matter of fact, people living in certain other societies almost never have heart attacks, because they eat, drink and live differently than most Americans.

Even if coronary artery disease has already started to develop in adults, lifestyle changes often can keep it from reaching the point where the person will suffer a heart attack or become disabled.

We can't guarantee that you will never have a heart attack if you read this book, but we can guarantee that you will have access to facts which may help you to prevent the disease. If you already suffer from atherosclerosis or coronary artery disease, many of the tips in this book may help you to keep your disease in check. Carefully consult with your own physician before using them. It can be dangerous to rely on self-diagnosis and self-treatment in cases of severe disease. Medical doctors have good success in treating patients with coronary artery disease, so talk to your physician and carefully follow his advice. Ask him if he thinks that some of the tips in this book may be helpful. Work with your doctor and not against him.

Heart Attacks, Coronary Artery Disease, Atherosclerosis — 20th Century Medical Problems Of Epidemic Proportions

<u>Heart Attack</u>!

An ambulance with a screaming siren speeds to the Emergency Room door of the hospital. Medics wheel the unconscious victim into the hospital on a stretcher. One medic presses on the victim's chest about once a second to compress his malfunctioning heart and keep the blood flowing, while another medic blows into his mouth every few seconds to keep his lungs inflated.

Finally, the victim reaches the coronary intensive care unit. There, doctors use electrical defibrillators to try to jolt the heart back into pumping on its own. Success! The victim's heart starts to beat again. The crisis is over. Slowly the sedated victim regains consciousness in a room in which he is wired to monitoring instruments and connected to tubes dispensing nutrients and drugs.

Prompt emergency care can save half of the victims of heart attacks. Many people are alive today because of quick medical response when they had a heart attack, but many others don't make it. Some survive one heart attack only to die after another one strikes. Coronary artery disease kills more people in our society than any other illness, but it doesn't have to be this way.

How Coronary Artery Disease Develops

Coronary artery disease starts when fatty streaks form in the inner linings of the *coronary arteries*, the arteries which feed blood to the heart muscle. Autopsies show that fatty streaks can begin in the main artery of the body, the *aorta*, actually in infancy. These buildups are frequently found in the smaller coronary arteries by the time children become teenagers. If the disease progresses, the fatty streaks may build up through the process of atherosclerosis into *atheromas*, which are small raised plaques of mushy cholesterol, fat and "foam cells" on the inner walls of the arteries. As the plaques grow, they may start to come together and seriously constrict the flow of blood within the arteries. Scar tissue may begin to grow under the fatty plaque, and this scar tissue may become "hardened" by deposits of calcium. Now the arteries have reached an advanced state of disease, and the flow of blood may be severely

6

constricted by hard, chalky plaque, which may not regress or shrink even with the best of care.

How A Heart Attack Happens

Heart attacks may happen after a piece of an atherosclerotic plaque comes loose and plugs a coronary artery, but many heart attacks happen without such a blockage or after a partial blockage from atherosclerosis upsets the rhythm of the heartbeat. During a heart attack, the heart may suddenly stop pumping blood effectively or go into a series of ineffective, twitching contractions called *fibrillation*. Fibrillation often can be stopped by an electrical shock given through the wall of the chest by an electronic defibrillator. After *defibrillation*, the heart may recover its normal beat.

The survival of a heart attack victim depends upon the severity of the attack and upon the swiftness of medical attention. Coronary intensive care units in major hospitals are well-equipped to handle heart attack emergencies, and a ride in a screaming ambulance to the hospital has saved many a life.

How To Tell If You're Having A Heart Attack

Some heart attacks are called *silent heart attacks*, because there is no advance warning. Many heart attacks are not unexpected, because the victim has suffered, perhaps for years, from *angina pectoris* or pain in the chest. Angina usually begins when progressive blocking of coronary arteries by atherosclerosis has reached an advanced stage that causes the heart to be starved for oxygen, because it isn't getting enough oxygen-carrying blood. Angina pectoris usually occurs after exertion, when the heart needs extra oxygen. It's a sudden pain or pressure in the chest behind the breastbone which may radiate down the shoulder, neck, arm, hand, or back, usually or mainly on the left side of the body. People with angina pectoris may also feel its sensations as being burning, choking, or feelings like indigestion.

If a heart attack is not occurring, angina usually will go away after a few minutes of rest or after the administration of doctor-prescribed *nitroglycerin*, which is taken as a tablet under the tongue to dilate or expand the coronary arteries. If angina lasts for more than five

8

minutes or if it is especially severe, it may be signalling the start of a heart attack, especially if it's accompanied by other symptoms, such as sweating or weakness. The type of angina which usually signals a heart attack is severe, lasts more than five minutes, is not completely relieved by stopping activity or administering nitroglycerin, and may be accompanied by sweating or weakness.

Here are the symptoms of having a heart attack:

1. heavy pressure or a choking or squeezing sensation in the center of the chest
2. chest pain which may radiate down one or both arms, across the back, or up the neck
3. shortness of breath
4. an unexplained sensation or feeling of fear
5. perspiration
6. nausea
7. dizziness or lightheadedness
8. weakness or a fainting sensation
9. angina pain that lasts for more than a few minutes or that doesn't go away upon administration of nitroglycerin and rest

All of these symptoms need not be present to indicate that a heart attack is taking place. Some can be caused by other problems, like indigestion.

Most heart attack victims who make it to the hospital will survive, but unfortunately, victims usually wait many hours before seeking medical help. Most people who die of heart attacks die outside the hospital. Knowledge of the symptoms of a heart attack and prompt action by calling an ambulance for a quick trip to the hospital can make the difference between life and death for a heart attack victim.

A Medical Mystery Solved — What Causes Atherosclerotic Artery Disease And Heart Attacks

Heart attacks are commonplace in the United States. They are so much on people's minds that whenever someone dies a sudden death, "heart attack" immediately comes to mind, but it was not always so.

Investigations of mummies from ancient China and ancient Egypt reveal that plaque sometimes could and did build up in the arteries of people in these ancient cultures.

Nevertheless, at the end of the 19th century, coronary artery disease in the United States was so *rare* that exact descriptions of it had not begun to be published. Dr. Paul Dudley White, the prominent cardiologist in the first half and middle of the 20th century who treated President Eisenhower after his heart attack, stated that he had never seen an autopsy of a heart attack victim until he was well into his years of practice.

What has caused this terrible epidemic of heart attacks — which kills fifty times as many Americans as the recently discovered AIDS epidemic? The answer becomes clear when we look at the changes which have taken place in our American way of life over the last one hundred years. These changes have been studied as *possible risk factors* — factors which can greatly increase our chances of developing artery disease and having heart attacks.

Researchers have studied populations of people who have low rates of heart attacks and compared them with peoples who have high rates of heart attacks. The differences in habits, customs, diets, environmental circumstances, heredity and other factors between such populations indicate that **artery disease is not** caused entirely by any one thing but by a multitude of factors, most of which are controllable if we know what they are and how to deal with them.

People in "primitive" cultures all around the world today have little artery disease and few heart attacks. People in "advanced" cultures like those in Europe and the United States have high rates of artery disease and frequent heart attacks. When people from rural areas in primitive countries move to big cities and adopt a westernized lifestyle, they soon start to suffer from coronary artery disease and other degenerative diseases to which their rural cousins are virtually immune. Similarly, when Japanese people, with their traditional rice and fish diet, move from Japan to Hawaii and change their diet and lifestyle, their rate of cardiovascular disease increases dramatically.

In World War II, people in countries like Austria experienced shortages of rich, high-fat foods like meat and cooking oil and substituted whole-grain products into their diets. During the shortages, the rate of heart attacks plummeted to low levels which had not been seen in those countries since the early 20th century.

Many risk factors which are presumed from geographical population studies have been confirmed by studying groups of individuals within larger populations: thin people vs. fat people, smokers vs. non-smokers, meat eaters vs. vegetarians, alcoholics vs. teetotalers, people with high blood pressure vs. people with low blood pressure, etc. Studies like these have reinforced theories which were developed after looking at populations in different cultures.

Finally, treatment programs designed to lower certain presumed risk factors have enjoyed some degree of success, even among people who have already started to develop artery disease. When people develop less atherosclerotic artery disease or have fewer heart attacks after undergoing a treatment program designed to lower one or more risk factors for the disease, the risk factor is well-proven. At that point, treatments based on lowering that risk factor will begin to be accepted among the medical community. Total lifestyle changes like those promoted at the Pritikin Centers and similar programs are many times more successful than attempts to peck away at risk factors.

Recently in the United States, the death rate from heart attacks and related artery disease has declined substantially, as more and more people have become aware that this disease is not inevitable. In fact, it is possible, if steps are taken early enough in a person's life, for the disease to become a *rarity* instead of almost a *certainty* as people age.

In the pages ahead, we want to tell you about the exciting new research findings of how the body cleans its own arteries, naturally! Then, we will examine well-established risk factors for this epidemic. We will also take a look at certain other risk factors which are possible contributors to the disease, although there isn't a large volume of research to "prove" or "disprove" how much these factors may contribute to artery disease. The final sections of this book will show how to take practical steps to reduce risk factors which are controllable.

But first, let's take a look at certain groups of people who are virtually free of heart and artery disease.

People Who Don't Get Heart Or Artery Disease

Are there individuals in our western culture who don't get heart or artery disease? Yes, there are such people, but isolated individuals within a population having similar lifestyles may only prove that certain people have a greater inherited resistance to the disease. What's important is that there are entire groups of people, all of whom are virtually free of heart and artery disease.

The New Guineans

One such artery disease-free group is the aboriginal natives of New Guinea. Researchers have made extensive studies of the New Guineans. They have discovered that of several hundred people who were examined, only two had even a mild case of angina pectoris; high blood pressure, stroke, and poor circulation in the legs were completely absent. Malnutrition, diabetes, obesity and other diseases that are commonplace in our culture were also absent.

Of course, the New Guineans were not perfectly healthy. Many suffered from respiratory diseases, worms and other parasites, and an unusual viral disease of the brain and nervous system (contracted by their cannibalistic practice of eating the brains of other human beings who were carriers of the disease).

The diet of the New Guineans at the time of the studies was composed almost entirely of sweet potatoes and sweet potato leaves, with less than 1% of their food coming from occasional barbecued pig feasts. Over 90% of their food was carbohydrate, mainly starch, with protein and fat each composing less than 5% of the diet. By our western dietary standards and the officially recommended daily dietary allowances for protein and fat, the New Guinea natives should have been severely malnourished, but they weren't. They retained enough protein from the very small amount in their diet to provide for not only the normal adult requirements, but also for the growth of children and the nourishment necessary for mothers to nurse their babies. The New Guinea natives were generally physically fit, trim and active. Their average protein intake for adults was only 20 grams per day, almost exclusively from plant protein sources which are generally considered to be deficient in certain key amino acids. (Comparatively, the average American consumes 100 grams or more of protein daily, mainly from animal sources.)

Tarahumara Indians

The Tarahumara Indians live in the Sierra Madre mountains in northern Mexico. Their diet and their lifestyle haven't been greatly changed by influences from outside their society, because of their isolation and travel customs. One of their interesting customs starts in early childhood, where boys and girls and men and women run for long distances playing a game of kickball as they run. Some of these races go on for days and cover as much as 200 miles from start to finish. During races, pulse rates rise to levels of 100 to 155, but blood pressure stays at a low level. These 50,000 Indians have no evidence of cardiovascular disease. None of the runners examined experience chest pain or shortness of breath during the races. None die from heart disease.

Some American long-distance runners drop dead of heart attacks, so the absence of artery disease among the Tarahumara Indians is surely also related to other factors besides running, such as their diet and perhaps, their drinking unchlorinated water. The diet of the Tarahumara Indians is made up mainly of high fiber corn meal. Carbohydrates account for about 80% of their caloric intake, with protein and fat each accounting for about 10%. Dietary fiber is very high, and nutritional deficiencies are rare.

In the 1970's, a few of the Tarahumara Indians were encouraged to participate in marathons in the U.S.A., but their finishing times were disappointing. This probably occurred because the long-distance races which they had been used to running (their "training") were conducted at paces of only 6 - 7 miles an hour while kicking and pursuing a ball. More specialized training, including practicing fast, steady, long runs, probably would have helped improve their performances.

The Inuit

The Inuit are a people living in the arctic circle, known to the outside world as Eskimos. Much of their ancient culture has disappeared in most Inuit communities because of air communication, trading posts, TV, alcohol, imported processed food, inactivity and other trappings of modern society. Fortunately, several Inuit communities were studied before these influences began to play a major role in their society.

The word "Eskimo" is an Algonquin Indian word for "eaters of raw flesh". Indeed, the Inuit do eat raw flesh. Much of their diet consists of fish, such as *char*, a red fleshed salmon-like fish of the Arctic Ocean. Wild game like caribou, musk-ox, seals, whales, birds and small mammals are also included in their diet. The Inuit also eat all parts of an animal: the bone marrow, the intestines, the internal organs and the fat.

The Inuit rarely eat regularly scheduled meals but instead snack on dried fish and game whenever they are hungry. Their food is dried without cooking. In hunting camps, game is community property, and everyone shares equally. Fasting and even starvation were not uncommon in Inuit society in earlier years, especially toward the end of winter when supplies ran low.

There are differences between the Inuit and other societies which are free from heart and artery disease. The Inuit diet is mostly protein and fat, like western diets; but there are unique aspects of their diet different from the high-fat, high-protein diets of western culture, which are proven to contribute to heart and artery disease. Fat in the Eskimo diet is not extremely high, being only perhaps 18% of total calories. Even more importantly, much of the fat in the Inuit diet is composed of fish oil, which is high in extremely unsaturated omega-3 fatty acids. Third, the fish and meat in the Inuit diet is not cooked but eaten raw, which leaves many nutrients and vitamins intact, such as vitamin B-6. Fourth, obesity is rare among Inuit living in a traditional wilderness culture. Finally, their drink is melted ice or snow or stream water.

The scientific community has criticized those studies of Inuit which show that there is very little heart disease among these people. One criticism is that the Inuit populations studied had very few old people in them. Therefore, just on the basis of age there should be little artery disease. Another criticism is that the methodology in the studies and the thoroughness of the examinations of the people studied was not rigorous.

In spite of these criticisms, there are two

major factors in the diet of the Inuit which have recently been discovered to be helpful in preventing artery disease. When food is cooked, it loses a large percentage of its natural vitamin content, including vitamin B-6; this particular vitamin actually helps protect the arteries against byproducts of protein metabolism, like homocysteine, which can cause artery damage and disease. So, eating raw meat and fish would preserve the natural vitamins. Secondly, cold water fish oil as a large part of the diet is apparently a great benefit in preventing artery disease, according to recent studies.

African Tribesmen

Rural African tribesmen are virtually free of coronary heart disease. Dr. Denis Burkitt, M.D., was the chief surgeon at the main hospital in Kampala, Uganda, for many years in the 1940's. Dr. Burkitt states that he saw approximately one case of angina pectoris per year and that coronary artery disease was virtually undetectable in the many autopsies he did each year. Dr. Burkitt says that over half of the people who died in the Kampala hospital were autopsied. The rare cases of coronary heart disease that he saw were in patients who

21

had adopted westernized patterns of diet and lifestyle in the urban area of Kampala. When Dr. Burkitt first started practicing in Africa, he was told by the head surgeon that he would probably never diagnose angina pectoris in an African who couldn't speak English, because that patient wouldn't have been affected by western diet.

African tribesmen typically eat a diet of mostly carbohydrates containing high levels of dietary fiber. Coarse ground corn meal is the main staple in the diet throughout much of Africa; other whole grain products and vegetables predominate in other areas where corn is not a staple. Meat composes a small percentage of the diet throughout most of rural Africa, with the exception of a few tribes such as the Masai, who are chiefly herdsmen.

Obesity is extremely rare among African tribesmen. This is quite a contrast to Americans of African descent who suffer from obesity just as much as do Americans of European descent. Dr. Burkitt states that the only obese Africans that he recalls having seen were those who had adopted westernized eating patterns.

Dr. Burkitt attributes the lack of coronary

artery disease among rural Africans to two major factors: first, the presence of vegetable fiber, primarily from whole grain sources in the diet; and secondly, the fact that the rural African diet is low in fat and sugar. Studies by Burkitt, Cleave, Heaton, Trowell and others indicate that digestion in people on a high-fiber diet takes place smoothly with the food moving quickly through the intestinal tract. Because of the rapid movement, cholesterol salts, excreted by the liver into the intestines, are swept away and eliminated. On a low-fiber western diet, however, the passage time of food through the intestines is slow, and constipation sets in; these same cholesterol-laden salts are reabsorbed into the bloodstream, leading to high levels of blood cholesterol and coronary heart disease. According to these physicians, the importance of dietary fiber in preventing coronary heart disease should not be underestimated. Also, according to these physicians, the absence of substantial amounts of sugar and fat in the diets of rural Africans is another significant factor in preventing coronary artery disease.

Summary — Things That People Who Are Virtually Free From Artery Disease Have In Common

Around the world, most populations which are virtually free of coronary artery disease share the following characteristics.

1) The drinking and cooking water is not chlorinated or artificially conditioned or softened.

2) Obesity is virtually non-existent.

3) With one exception, the Inuit, the main staples in the diet are whole grains or vegetable products with minimal processing which are low in protein, extremely low in fat, and high in dietary fiber.

4) Exercise is a part of everyday life.

5) The Inuit, who eat a diet which is high in protein and moderate in fat, consume their protein in an uncooked form, and much of their fat intake is fish oil, which contains omega-3 fatty acids.

These characteristics of peoples who are virtually free from coronary artery disease will become especially meaningful in later chapters as we examine *risk factors*. Attempts to combat coronary artery disease by reducing some, but not all, of the risk factors which are controllable have met with mixed success. Such attempts generally have shown *some* reduction in rates of coronary artery disease. Steps to reduce risk factors usually do not produce dramatic results unless *most* of the above characteristics are closely mimicked.

Some of the above characteristics are not generally recognized as being proven risk factors. Chlorination of water supplies is one such neglected area. Water chlorination is proven to increase the rates of certain kinds of cancer, but there have been no thorough studies showing whether it does or does not increase the rate of artery disease or heart attacks. By the same token, the consumption of large amounts of cooked meat containing animal fat is proven to be a risk factor for developing coronary artery disease; but there has been no adequate research to show definitely if the consumption of large amounts of uncooked meat, as in the Inuit, removes or lessens the risk of artery disease from such consumption.

Proven Risk Factors Which M
Or Contribute To The Devel
Coronary Artery Disease
Attacks

Smoking: The Single, Most Preventable Cause of Heart Disease

Like most people, you are probably aware that smoking is bad for your health. Tobacco has been linked to many diseases including Alzheimer's Disease, heart and blood vessel disorders, cancer, emphysema, bronchitis, asthma, birth defects and low-birth weights in infants of women who smoked during pregnancy. Cigarette smoking is believed to account for over one-third of all deaths from heart disease. The American Heart Association states that "smoking is the single *most preventable* cause of these diseases and deaths from them."

Chemicals of Smoking — The nicotine in cigarettes causes addiction to smoking. Doctors report that nicotine from an inhaled cigarette reaches the brain in seven seconds, twice as fast as it does in an intravenous injection. At the rate of 10 puffs per cigarette, a one pack a day smoker gets over 70,000 "shots" of nicotine per year.

27

Nicotine is a deadly poison. One drop of pure nicotine in solution will kill a human being instantly. Diluted, it is used commercially for killing insects. Nicotine in less than lethal doses strains the heart by constricting blood vessels, making it hard for the blood to flow through them. This raises blood pressure and increases heart rate.

Furthermore, cigarette smoke causes certain glands in the body to release adrenalin and other hormones. Adrenalin speeds up the heartbeat. Carbon monoxide, found in cigarette smoke, is the same poisonous gas found in automobile exhaust. Carbon monoxide in a closed area can suffocate and kill. It combines easily with the hemoglobin in red blood cells and replaces some of the oxygen carried by the blood, because it has a greater attraction to hemoglobin than oxygen.

The level of carbon monoxide in a smoker's blood can be as much as 15 times higher than in a non-smoker. It stays in the bloodstream as long as six hours after smoking. Although levels of carbon monoxide found in the blood after smoking aren't high enough to kill smokers directly, such levels may have a slightly negative effect on attentiveness and the ability to think. Elevated levels of carbon monoxide may also damage the arteries or increase the rate at which cholesterol is deposited on the inner walls of the arteries.

Besides nicotine and carbon monoxide, tobacco contains tar. Cigarette tar is transformed into a vapor as cigarettes are smoked. Cigarette tar is composed of thousands of different chemicals. One-third of these chemicals are carcinogens, cancer causing substances. The respiratory system of the smoker becomes lined with sticky black tar, making it difficult to breathe. Cilia in the lungs are microscopic, hair-like bristles which sweep up and out, pushing mucus, germs and dirt out of the lungs and bronchial tubes. Smoking even one cigarette slows down this function, and heavy smoking destroys the cilia, resulting in "smoker's cough".

Low-tar cigarettes aren't necessarily better than regular cigarettes. They contain less nicotine, so the smoker may inhale more often to get a stronger nicotine "fix", and he may actually take in more tar and other poisons. This may nullify the claimed benefits of low-tar brands.

Even the choices of over 1,400 different flavoring ingredients may be harmful when combined with the other chemicals in cigarettes.

Smoking just one cigarette speeds up the heartbeat, increases blood pressure, decreases lung capacity and causes a drop in the skin temperature of fingers and toes. Smoking also diminishes the sense of taste and smell. Even early aging of the skin can be attributed to smoking because it causes wrinkles by constricting blood vessels and reducing vitamin C levels in the skin, which helps keep it supple and elastic. Sugar in cigarette tar can cause tooth decay.

The American Lung Association has found that the smoke which drifts away from the burning end of a cigarette contains more harmful substances than the smoke inhaled from the other end of the cigarette by the smoker. The smoke from just two cigarettes an hour in a room accumulates to an amount greater than that considered safe by the Environmental Protection Agency. In one study, children exposed to smoke in a small room for 30 minutes showed an increase in heart rate and blood pressure, as well as a rise in the level of carbon monoxide in their blood. Other effects of the "accidental" inhalation of smoke while being in a room with smoke in it include eye and throat irritation, respiratory and circulatory symptoms and even an increased risk of throat cancer. One study shows that non-smokers who live in a house with a smoker have one and a half times the rate of heart attacks that other non-smokers have.

History of Smoking — Every known variety of tobacco plant was originally found in North and South America. The Mayan Indians of Mexico were the first to burn tobacco and inhale smoke. Thousands of years ago, the Mayans believed tobacco smoke could keep away evil winds and poisonous snakes, protect night travelers and those who worked in dark places, cure illness, protect an unborn child and rid a dwelling of ghosts and evil spirits. Smoking became a tribal ritual for the American Indians, and Christopher Columbus reported that the Indians "drank the smoke of curious dried leaves". He took tobacco seeds back to Europe, and it wasn't long before smoking was an established habit. Sir Walter Raleigh, the famous English explorer, became a smoker soon after he visited the New World. There is a story that when his servant first saw him smoking, he thought Raleigh was on fire and quickly splashed a bucket of water over him.

As early as 1575, Mexican priests were instructed by their council to forbid smoking in the church, and in 1642 Pope Urban VIII issued a formal bill against tobacco. Pope Innocent X did the same in 1650. King James I of England realized some of the health hazards of smoking when he stated in 1604 that smoking is a "custom loathsome to the eye, hateful to the nose, harmful to the brain, dangerous to the lungs..."

It wasn't until the 1920's that doctors and scientists began to investigate extensively the effects of smoking on our general health.

Health Hazard Reports of Smoking — The American Cancer Society issued its first warning in 1954 that "Cigarette smoking is the major known cause in lung cancer deaths." The United States' Surgeon General's Reports of 1964 and 1979 have helped convince one million people a year to quit smoking, and the majority of people who smoke wish they had never started.

The Federal Trade Commission ruled in 1967 that the "Fairness Doctrine" that had been applied to political campaigns should also apply to cigarette advertising. In other words, the advertisers had to give equal time to warnings on the risks of smoking. Paradoxically, putting this warning on cigarette packages and cigarette advertising has probably saved the tobacco companics from bankruptcy by lawsuits from people who have died from the effects of smoking. The task force appointed by the Surgeon General in 1968 stated that the tobacco industry was "encouraging death and disease", and in 1971, the United States was the twelfth country to ban cigarette advertising from radio and television.

The 1979 Surgeon General's Report shows that smoking is far more dangerous than was indicated in the first report in 1964. The following immediate effects of tobacco have been observed in smokers: circulation in the fingers and toes decreases, the heart muscle works harder to consume more oxygen, blood pressure rises, heart rhythms become irregular, and there may be other changes in the electrical activity, as measured by the electrocardiograph (EKG) machine. Scientists believe these effects may be due to the release of nerve-stimulating hormones from the adrenal glands lying over the kidneys. The effects of nicotine are similar to those of other stimulants, which may be why some smokers feel more alert after smoking, although there are no controlled experiments to prove this theory.

Results of Smoking — After years of research, long-term effects of smoking on the heart and arteries are now known. The Veterans Administration Hospitals reported in 1976 that autopsies revealed coronary artery disease to be 4.4 times more common in those who smoked two packs or more of cigarettes per day than in non-smokers. Population studies indicate that there is an association between cigarette smoking and an increase in the incidence of heart attacks. The reason heart attacks occur usually is attributed to an increase in fatty deposits and hardening of the heart's arteries, both hazards of smoking, which result in less blood supply to the heart muscle.

Smoking acts together with high blood pressure and elevated blood cholesterol to increase the chances of a heart attack occurring. A five-year study published in the *American Heart Journal* (May, 1977) showed that the number of cigarettes smoked daily correlates with the occurrence of a heart attack among men who have had prior attacks. In a Swedish study reported in 1977, men who quit smoking after their first attack had only half the rate of fatal and nonfatal heart attacks as those who continued to smoke over a two-year follow-up period.

Smoking may also increase the risk of stroke. The majority of strokes are classified either as brain hemorrhage associated with high blood pressure or more commonly, cutoff of blood to the brain associated with blood clots of the vessels of the neck and their main branches in the brain that diminish the supply of blood to the brain. A recent study of a large group of women reported that cigarette smoking when combined with the use of oral contraceptives (the pill) increases the risk of brain hemorrhage 22 times.

Smoking can directly raise blood pressure. However, there is conflicting evidence about whether or not smoking induces chronic hypertension. Some studies report that the incidence of hypertension is greater in smokers while others report that smokers actually have slightly lower blood pressure than nonsmokers. On the whole, studies indicate that smoking is not a major contributor to hypertension; but when high blood pressure is present, in combination with other risk factors, such as elevated blood fats, smoking makes things worse.

Smoking also can contribute to atherosclerotic *peripheral vascular disease* (PVD), a narrowing or blocking of the leg arteries. Studies on people without cardiovascular disease showed a decreased blood flow to the arms and legs when tested during smoking. Heavy smokers who stopped smoking, however, showed an increase in blood flow to the arms and legs during the time they stopped. Smoking greatly increases the risk of PVD in diabetics.

Rupture of the *aorta*, the largest artery in the body, after it balloons out in an aortic *aneurysm*, has been associated with smoking. The aorta is the main channel of the arterial system, the great vessel that arches from the top of the heart and passes down through the chest and abdomen. Two extensive research studies found a direct correlation between the amount of cigarettes smoked and death from rupture of the aorta. The mortality rate of a pack-a-day man was four or five times normal, whereas it was seven and eight times normal for a man who smokes two packs a day. Carbon monoxide exposure may create conditions that promote plaque growth and lack of oxygen which harm the aorta, or smoking may lead to excessive blood clot formation, which in turn leads to excessive plaque formation and aneurysms.

Many studies have shown that smokers have somewhat higher blood cholesterol levels than nonsmokers, but the differences have been too small to account for the observed differences in risk associated with smoking. Smoking and high cholesterol are considered two independent risk factors.

Cigarette smoking is a proven risk factor for cardiovascular disease. It is not a necessary condition for them, since hardening of the arteries and heart attacks do occur in nonsmokers. However, extensive research shows that smoking in the absence of increases in other risk factors is sufficient to increase mortality from heart attacks.

More than 200,000 Americans die prematurely each year from cardiovascular diseases because they smoked. The good news is that people who stop smoking have their risk of cardiovascular disease revert to nonsmokers' levels after 10 years. A heavy smoker can add 6 to 10 years to his life expectancy by quitting. Most of this increase in life expectancy is from a reduction in rates of heart and artery disease, but many other diseases are combatted by giving up smoking.

Cigarette smokers are at an increased risk for respiratory tract infections. It has been shown that smokers have more influenza than nonsmokers. Bronchitis and emphysema are also related to cigarette smoking, as is lung cancer, which was a rare disease just 50 years ago. Today, it is the number one cancer killer among men. Furthermore, a study on children aged 10 to 12 who admitted smoking at least one cigarette per day showed that they exhibited respiratory symptoms.

Smoking cigarettes is also related to cancer of the digestive system, including oral cancer, cancer of the esophagus and cancer of the pancreas. Smoking may also be directly related to the development of gastric and duodenal ulcers, and it may retard the healing of the ulcers.

Smoking is one of the chief causes of hiatal hernia and heartburn. Apparently, smoking loosens the tension of the esophageal sphincter muscle that keeps stomach acid out of the esophagus and throat. Smokers frequently have burning sensations in the throat and chest from heartburn.

There is a strong association between cigarette smoking and cancer of the urinary bladder in men and women and cancer of the kidney in men. Cigarette smoking probably acts together with other risk factors, such as occupational exposure to amine dyes and the ingestion of saccharin, to cause bladder cancer. On the average, cigarette smokers are twice as likely to die from cancer of the bladder as are nonsmokers.

Cigarette smoking during pregnancy has an adverse effect not only upon the well-being of the pregnant woman, but on the developing fetus, newborn infant and growing child. Low birth weight of infants, bleeding due to placental problems and hemorrhage in the latter half of pregnancy are hazards to both mother and baby. Most smoking-related birth defects are multiple and major and kill very early, usually before delivery of the child. Smoking during pregnancy can also be related to miscarriage, premature births and congenital malformations. After birth, infants of smokers seem to have higher rates of respiratory illnesses, like bronchitis and pneumonia, during the first year of life.

Men who smoke have a reduction in

proportion of active sperm, directly related to the number of cigarettes smoked. The incidence of deformed sperm in smokers is significantly greater, possibly causing birth defects and infertility.

Doctors have long noted the association between the development or aggravation of allergies or allergy symptoms and direct exposure to tobacco and tobacco products. Allergies were not reviewed in the 1964 Surgeon General's Report, but studies in the late 1960s and 1970s indicate that tobacco and its smoke can affect the immune system in one of two ways: by interacting with the immune system to produce an allergic response, or by interacting with the special cells of the immune system, influencing these natural defenders to function improperly. Studies indicate that younger smokers may be at greater risk of suffering heart attacks than older smokers because of allergies to tobacco smoke. Repeated exposure to the allergens in cigarette smoke may cause accelerated cardiovascular disease and higher death rates.

Tobacco smoke contains thousands of substances, many of which act directly on the body and others that interact with other chemicals, like prescription drugs, taken into the body. The clinical effects of smoking may include accelerated rates of drug processing in the body, decreased intensity and duration of drugs' effects, in other words causing decreased therapeutic benefits derived from drugs.

In some cases, the effects of smoking are so dramatic that interpreting medical test results without taking into consideration the patient's smoking history could lead to an incorrect diagnosis or inappropriate treatment.

Some people are more vulnerable to the physical effects of tobacco smoke — unborn infants, children, workers in the asbestos, rubber, coal, textile, uranium and chemical industries and all those with family medical histories of heart, lung or malignant diseases. Since World War I, women have been smoking more. The gap between men and women for heart attacks and sudden cardiac death has narrowed in recent years.

In his foreward to the Surgeon General's Report of 1979, former secretary of the Department of Health, Education and Welfare, Joseph A. Califano, Jr., stated: "Today there can be no doubt that smoking is truly slow-motion suicide".

41

Giving Up Smoking — Using other tobacco products may be less harmful, overall, than smoking cigarettes, but smoking cigars, pipes and chewing smokeless tobacco greatly increases risks for cancer of the throat, mouth, tongue and neck.

Most people can't give up smoking without determination and help from everyone who cares for the smoker. Withdrawal from nicotine can be eased by a prescription drug called Nicorette® which slowly releases a measured dose of nicotine into the system to reduce physical craving for tobacco products. Withdrawal from nicotine may also be eased by taking half a teaspoon of bicarbonate of soda in a glass of water two or three times a day. Apparently, the bicarbonate of soda helps hold nicotine in the system and reduce withdrawal symptoms by giving the body more time to adapt to withdrawal.

Once a smoker has successfully withdrawn from tobacco for two weeks, most withdrawal symptoms should pass.

Regular aerobic exercise such as running, walking, playing tennis, swimming, bike riding, hard physical labor and association with nonsmokers help smokers to quit and to resist temptation to return to smoking.

Air Pollution

Death rates, including deaths from heart attacks, rise when smog attacks a city. The elderly are hit much harder than younger people, since smog puts a strain on weak hearts and lungs. Carbon monoxide, a component of the pollution from automobile exhaust, can starve the heart of oxygen and even trigger an attack of angina pectoris for those who drive on crowded highways.

Even so, city-wide air pollution is probably a small risk factor when compared with localized air pollution from cigarette smoke. Living in the same house with a smoker or working in an office where people smoke puts a person at more risk than living in a city with extremely high air pollution at the peak of the smog season.

Lack of Exercise

Many research studies have established the relationship between lack of exercise and increased risk of coronary heart disease or heart attacks. One of the first studies was among active and inactive workers in London. Researchers found that the city's bus drivers, who sat down all day, had 30 percent more heart attacks than the conductors on the same buses, who ran up and down the double-decker buses collecting fares. In the United States, researchers kept records of thousands of railroad clerks and switchmen for 10 years and found that the less active clerks had a 20 percent greater incidence of coronary heart disease than the more active clerks. Another study showed that American automobile factory foremen had more heart attacks than the workers they supervised who got more exercise on the job. A recent study shows that older people with painful foot problems, which prevented normal standing or walking, had higher than expected rates of heart attacks.

Aerobic exercise is one of the most beneficial forms of exercise and one of the most efficient ways of getting in shape. Aerobic activities such as swimming, dancing, running or jogging, cycling or brisk walking strengthen your cardiovascular system by demanding oxygen. A heart that has been strengthened by exercise beats fewer times per minute to supply the body's oxygen needs, functions at a lower blood pressure and requires less oxygen for itself. Exercise also improves respiration. The lungs are able to take in more air and deliver oxygen to the tissues more efficiently.

Even moderate, low-key exercise may help reduce heart disease risk. A study of over 4,000 Californians showed that those who took stairs instead of the elevator or walked instead of driving had lower blood pressure and less body fat than less active people.

Unaccustomed, Strenuous Exercise or Sudden Stopping of Exercise

While many studies show that regular, sustained aerobic exercise strengthens the heart, unaccustomed bursts of exercise can sometimes precipitate a heart attack. Running races, especially races ending with sprints, running hard in the morning instead of later in the day, running on cold days, running on hot days, shoveling snow or working hard outdoors on cold days and other forms of sudden exercise or hard, unaccustomed work, especially in cold or very hot weather, can lead to heart attacks in susceptible people. "Warming up" and "cooling down" gradually is advised to reduce risk whenever exercising strenuously.

According to tradition, in 490 B.C., the Greek runner Pheidippides ran more than 26 miles from the plain of Marathon to Athens to deliver the news to his countrymen that their army had defeated the Persians. Only minutes after delivering the good news, he dropped dead. Doctors think now that "post-exercise sudden death" is caused by a buildup of two stress hormones during strenuous exercise which continue to increase after exercise. A cool-down period after vigorous exercise is recommended to allow the body to gradually lower its level of activity.

One of the authors personally witnessed the death of a long-distance runner after a 5 kilometer race. The runner was a lean, physically fit man in his fifties who had run several much longer marathon races and who had climbed mountains in the Alps.

It was a clear but cold morning in Montreal on the day of the race, and the man who was to die within the hour was late for the race. As the starter's gun sounded, the runner who was late for the race displayed signs of anger at the registration table, and then he took off in a hurry after the pack of racers. He passed me at the half-mile mark at a rate of speed which, if continued, probably would have won the race.

When I finished the race, I saw him sprawled out over a brick planter in the hotel lobby. All attempts to revive him failed.

The late runner did several things which increased his risk in running.

1) He was angry, and anger increases the tendency of the blood to clot.

2) He was running on a cold morning. Cold weather increases the chances of blood clots forming or of the heart going into a spasm. Also, heart attacks in runners are more likely to happen in the morning than during other times of the day.

3) He ran without warming up.

4) In his efforts to catch up with the field, he was probably running too fast for his ability.

The tragedy that I witnessed was sobering, and I'm hoping that its relation here in these pages will encourage people who exercise strenuously to take proper precautions and to have a balanced mental attitude, which is not overly competitive, towards running or other sports.

Alcoholism

Alcoholism is an addiction to the drug alcohol, sometimes referred to as "the most abused drug in the United States." As a nation, we spend more money on alcohol than we do on our health. It is a definite risk factor which leads to high blood pressure, increased heart attacks, cirrhosis of the liver, serious diseases of the stomach, and may actually cause the brain to shrink.

Recent studies indicate that moderate consumption of alcohol, arbitrarily set at one ounce or less of alcohol per day, especially in the form of beer or wine, may not increase the risk of artery disease or heart attack. Some researchers think that moderate consumption of alcohol may reduce the chances of developing coronary artery disease in people who don't get regular, aerobic exercise. However, most physicians do not think this conclusion is warranted, and that more studies are needed.

Research shows that the consumption of

alcohol, even in moderation, increases risk factors by reducing glucose or sugar tolerance, raising blood pressure and increasing body weight. Moderate consumption of alcoholic beverages can lead to alcoholism, accidents and other alcohol-related diseases.

Heredity and Other Uncontrollable Risk Factors

Some risks can't be controlled; but, when an uncontrollable risk factor is present, extra care can be taken to minimize other risks which can be controlled. People who come from families where their parents or other close relatives have had coronary artery disease are at greater risk than people who come from families with low rates. Age is a factor. Four out of five deaths in America from heart attacks occur after age 65, but in some parts of the world, the incidence of heart attacks, strokes and other atherosclerosis-related diseases in the elderly is low. Therefore, cardiovascular disease is not an inevitable part of aging.

The differences in male and female hormones are also factors. Under age 60, twice as many men as women have heart attacks, but the difference evens out over the age of 65. Premenopausal women have significantly lower rates of coronary artery disease than men. However, as women's lifestyles change, increased risk may result. Women are smoking more, working at high-powered, stressful jobs, getting less exercise and taking birth control pills, all of which increase their risk of artery disease.

Increased risk is noted if an electrocardiogram taken after a resting period is normal shows abnormal readings when taken after exercise.

Heredity and other uncontrollable risk factors explain why some people may suffer from coronary artery disease even though they practice preventive measures, while others may get away with poor health practices and never develop heart disease. To further complicate matters, many "macho" men, consciously or unconsciously, may deny problems or resist therapy. Not admitting their personal vulnerability may result in an early or dramatic death.

Diabetes

Diabetes is a great risk factor for artery disease. Dr. James Anderson's work on lowering blood sugar and LDL cholesterol levels with a high-starch, high-fiber, low-sugar, moderate-calorie diet, which is reported a few pages later, is of great interest to diabetics. He has written a book on the subject, *Diabetes*, that should be must reading for adult onset diabetics and their physicians.

Being Overweight

It's true that most Americans live to eat rather than eat to live. People who are above average weight for their age and height are more likely to have heart attacks than people who are close to normal weight. The more overweight a person is, the more likely he is to have a heart attack because of more strain on the heart and circulatory system. The extra weight a person carries is adipose (fat) tissue, which must be serviced by capillaries like the rest of the body.

Even a person 15 pounds overweight has millions of extra capillaries putting a strain on the heart. Obese people may suffer from increased rates of coronary artery disease because of being overweight, having a greater tendency toward diabetes, or because of diet. Compared with a person of normal weight, the overweight person's chances of developing high blood pressure are three to four times greater; for developing diabetes, four to five times greater; and for coronary heart disease, two or three times.

Obesity is a social problem. Look at any women's magazine, and you'll see thin models and articles on health and fitness, yet recipes with pictures of fattening, unhealthy foods. The use of sugar in beverages, cakes, ice cream, jelly and in less obvious foods, such as pickles and cured bacon, has skyrocketed to the point where an average American may eat as much as 100 pounds of sugar a year. With meats, butter, milk and other fatty foods being plentiful, Americans tend to eat too much food and the wrong kinds of food. And most of America's food budget goes for processed foods rather than natural, nutritious ones.

There are several popular misconceptions as to why American adults are overweight. One blames an underactive thyroid gland, or hypothyroidism, which causes people with this condition to gain weight more readily than someone with a normally functioning thyroid. Although this is a real condition, it is not common and is easily diagnosed and readily treated. Another misconception is too many fat cells. Studies have shown that people who have been overweight from childhood have a normal number of fat cells but an abnormal amount of fat in those cells. These people can achieve normal weight. Sometimes laziness is blamed, although laziness is usually a result of being overweight rather than the cause. It takes more effort for a fat person to move. They feel and look clumsy and often experience feelings of low self-esteem.

What is responsible for obesity in most people? — the abnormal diet that most Americans daily consume. Another factor in obesity is lack of understanding of food values, calorie content and nutritional benefits. Emotions play a part, too. People who are anxious, tense, insecure or angry turn to food as a release. Food can also become a substitute for a feeling of well-being, comfort, contentment or loneliness. We condition ourselves to eat what, where, how much and when we eat. Some people eat while watching TV, driving the car, studying, reading, preparing a meal or before going to bed at night.

You *can* change your behavior. You *can* say no to old habits and stop making excuses for them or even blaming others.

High-Salt Diets

High blood pressure is a risk factor which is associated with coronary artery disease. If a person has coronary artery disease, high blood pressure increases the risk. High blood pressure, especially, increases the risk of stroke which is related to artery disease.

Salt, or sodium chloride, is essential to life. It is an important mineral in the body without which we would all die. In the Bible, Jesus says, "Ye are the salt of the earth", indicating that even thousands of years ago salt was a valuable commodity for preserving food and stimulating taste buds. In the Roman army, the word from which we get our word "salary" was the Latin work "sal", meaning salt. Roman soldiers were sometimes said to be "worth their salt" because they were often paid in salt rather than actual money.

Salt has come a long way since ancient times. Today it's inexpensive and is the most frequently used seasoning and preservative. Sodium, part of the sodium chloride salt molecule, is also found in other forms. Technically, it is the sodium in salt that is the gremlin (bad factor), but we will use "salt" as a more common term.

The average American eats five to ten grams, or as much as one third of an ounce, of salt per day. This is much more salt than is needed for bodily functions. Recent studies indicate that some people need as little as one-fifth of a gram (200 milligrams) of sodium per day. However, there are exceptions: hard labor, hot weather, pregnancy and breast-feeding may increase the need for sodium up to 2 grams per day.

Most people will question whether they really consume one-third to one-fifth of an ounce of salt per day, but processed foods that Americans eat are usually filled with salt. Any food that comes in a can, frozen packet or a box is likely to have salt added as a preservative or flavor enhancer.

A typical slice of bread may contain over 200 milligrams (mg.) of salt, a bowl of corn flakes over 300 mg., a bowl of canned soup over 1,000 mg., a TV dinner over 2,500 mg., a chicken dinner from a fast food restaurant over 2,000 mg., and a large dill pickle over 1,000 mg.

Scientific studies indicate that salt preference is a learned habit — an acquired taste. As people reduce the amount of salt in their diets, they experience new flavor sensations which were masked by large amounts of salt they used to eat. The true flavor of vegetables can be hidden by cooking with too much salt. In this sense, excessive salt can be a taste-destroyer rather than a flavor enhancer.

One scientific study on salt consumption deals with twins. One twin is put on a low-salt diet. The other twin continues to consume a diet high in salt. After a few weeks, the twin on the low-salt diet has learned to consume less salt and prefers to eat less salt. The other twin is still in the habit of consuming more salt and continues to prefer the high-salt diet.

Many scientific studies show that reducing salt intake will lower blood pressure in most people by a significant amount. Getting salt intake down in the range of 500 mg. of salt per day helps the most. Reducing salt intake lowers blood pressure dramatically in some people who have a tendency toward high blood pressure; thus, the benefits of reduced salt consumption are greater for some of the people who need the benefits the most, those with life and threatening high blood pressure.

Studies around the world show that the more salt a particular society consumes, the greater the number of cases of severe high blood pressure. It is significant that the Greenland Eskimos, who eat very little salt, have very little high blood pressure, but in the north of Japan, high blood pressure is common among the people whose diet contains large amounts of salt.

Statistics show that high blood pressure occurs more commonly in people who salt their food before tasting it than in people who taste their food first and add salt only if necessary. Reducing salt intake to very low levels sometimes will help reduce high blood pressure in people who are salt sensitive.

Hypertension (High Blood Pressure)

High blood pressure is a dangerous disease. An estimated 60 million Americans have some form of hypertension, yet up to half of these victims are unaware that they have the disease. It is a subtle condition, often with no obvious symptoms in its early stages, yet hypertensive people are three to five times more vulnerable to heart attack than those with normal blood pressure.

Blood pressure is the force exerted on the walls of arteries, veins and capillaries as the heart pumps blood through the body. Without enough pressure, blood would not be able to pick up oxygen from the lungs or force impurities through the kidneys to the bladder. Blood pressure is taken with an arm pressure cuff in two readings: for example, 120/80. The first number refers to systolic pressure, or the pressure which is produced as the heart contracts to pump blood out into the body. The second number is diastolic pressure, the pressure which remains in the blood vessels as the heart relaxes to allow for the flow of blood into its pumping chambers. The most accurate way to measure blood pressure is sitting down with your arm resting on a table level with your heart.

"Normal" blood pressure readings are based on average blood pressures for different age groups. Temporary hypertension is a normal rise in blood pressure to meet the body's needs in times of stress or increased bodily activity, such as digestion or exercise. But, regardless of age, high blood pressure above 140/90 which is sustained for a long period of time, will damage the body and should be treated by a physician who hopefully won't ignore natural methods which can work with cooperative patients.

High blood pressure can damage the interior and exterior arteries. It can also damage key organs, such as the brain, heart and kidneys. Persistent high blood pressure can also cause stroke or heart attack. A stroke occurs when blood vessels become blocked and cut off the flow of blood to the brain, or when blood vessels break and allow blood to leak into brain tissue. It may take years for high blood pressure to weaken and damage blood vessels, but a stroke can happen within seconds with no warning. With most heart attacks, the small coronary arteries become blocked and stop part or all of the heart from pumping blood. High blood pressure can also place an extra burden on the heart, which in time will cause the heart to weaken. Fluid builds up in the body's tissues and kidneys may fail. Congestive heart failure occurs when fluid has built up around the heart and chokes it.

The major contributor to high blood

pressure is salt, or sodium chloride. It is an essential mineral in the body, but used in excess in flavoring and as a preservative. Heavy metals such as cadmium and lead, found in small trace amounts in water supplies in the United States may also contribute to high blood pressure. Caffeine is another major contributor. It is found in most cola drinks, coffee, tea and chocolate. Smog and tobacco smoke are also significant in raising blood pressure. Lack of exercise will make the heart become weak, resulting in more work for the heart to pump. High-fat diets can cause hardening of the arteries which leads to high blood pressure. And excessive alcohol drinking, more than one ounce per day, not only raises blood pressure, but damages the liver and kidneys, as well.

High-Fat Diets

For many years, medical researchers have warned against diets that are high in fat as being a factor that leads to coronary artery disease. Over the years, the case has become stronger against high-fat diets, especially diets which are high in saturated fat. Saturated fats raise the blood cholesterol and triglyceride levels. They are primarily found in animal and dairy products such as fats in meats, egg yolks, milk, butter, cheese, cream and a few vegetable fats, such as coconut oil and hydrogenated vegetable shortenings. Saturated fats are generally hard or solid at room temperature.

On the other hand, polyunsaturated fats help to lower the level of cholesterol in the blood. They are mostly derived from plant and vegetable sources, such as cottonseed, soybean, corn and safflower. Sunflower and sesame seeds, walnuts and pecans are also high in polyunsaturates. Polyunsaturated fats are usually soft or liquid at room temperature.

Studies show that in the United States and other countries where the typical diet is high in meat, dairy fats, refined and processed foods, there are high blood-cholesterol levels, atherosclerosis and a high heart attack rate. But in countries such as Japan and Yugoslavia where more fruit, vegetables, fish and cereal grains are eaten, cholesterol levels and coronary disease levels are significantly lower.

Other research shows that groups of people within certain countries, such as Seventh Day Adventists in the United States who generally have low-fat, mostly vegetarian diets, have substantially lower rates of coronary artery disease than their neighbors, who come from the same background, but who eat foods high in fat like those of the typical American diet.

Other studies show that when meat and dairy products and total food calories are in short supply, as they were in many European countries during World War II, the rate of coronary heart attack was lowered. For example, in Austria toward the end of the war, the heart attack rate was only 12% of the pre-war heart attack rate. After the war was over, Austrians resumed their old dietary habits and the rate of heart attacks soon increased to pre-war levels.

Current studies indicate that a wise, low-fat diet can not only lower blood cholesterol and help prevent atherosclerosis, but may be able to help combat atherosclerosis where it already exists.

Occasionally a researcher will argue that the case against high-fat diets is not completely proven, because high-fat diets may be linked to other factors such as Western lifestyle, high amounts of protein in the diet, lack of dietary fiber or high amounts of salt in the diet. While it is true that other factors may also contribute to coronary artery disease, the evidence is quite strong that high saturated fat diets are a major factor leading to coronary artery disease.

High Blood Cholesterol

High levels of cholesterol in the blood are a risk factor for coronary artery disease. One of the most interesting facts that has been discovered in recent years is the process by which arteries become narrowed and finally clogged up with deposits, including cholesterol.

Cholesterol is a fatty, waxy substance found only in animal products. Most of it found in the human body is produced in the liver, but 20 to 30 percent is derived from the food we eat. Despite its bad reputation, cholesterol is essential to life. It is a building block of the outer membrane of cells, and a principal ingredient in the digestive juice, bile. It is present in the fatty sheath that insulates nerves. It's a precursor of the steroid hormones, including the sex hormones. The ideal cholesterol level is below 200 mg. Average levels for Americans are 200-240 mg. Levels above 240 mg. are considered to be elevated. Populations who arc virtually free of artery disease usually have cholesterol levels of 150 mg. or lower.

Medical researchers have discovered that cholesterol and other fats are carried in different forms in the bloodstream in several protein-fat combinations, called lipoproteins. The two major types of lipoproteins are *high density lipoproteins* (HDL's) and *low density lipoproteins* (LDL's). HDL's, the "good" cholesterol, help remove cholesterol from circulation, thus reducing the risk of heart disease; LDL's, the "bad" cholesterol, circulate in the blood, depositing fat and cholesterol in the tissues, forming a major part of a build-up in the artery wall. Studies have shown that the higher the level of LDL's, the greater the risk of coronary heart disease, but the higher the level of HDL's, the lower the risk of coronary heart disease.

As early as 1913, Russian Pathologist Nikolai Anitschkow showed that he could produce cholesterol deposits, or plaques, in the arteries of rabbits just by feeding them a cholesterol-rich diet. In 1947, a study of seven nations showed a direct relationship between a country's incidence of heart disease, the level of cholesterol in the blood and the amount of animal fat in the national diet. The Finns, with the diet highest in fat, had the highest cholesterol levels and the highest rate of heart disease; Americans had the second highest cholesterol levels and second highest rate of heart disease. But in Japan, where diets were low in fat, the cholesterol levels were the lowest and heart disease was the least.

Atherosclerosis, hardening of the arteries, can actually begin in youth. A study revealed that 77 percent of American soldiers killed in the Korean War were found in autopsies to have hardening of the arteries. The average age of the soldiers was 22 years. The arteries of the opposing young Korean soldiers of comparable age, whose diets were rice and vegetables, showed no atherosclerosis. The results of autopsies were much the same during the Vietnamese war.

Cholesterol-rich foods, such as eggs, organ meats and most cheeses may directly contribute to high levels of potentially harmful LDL's. Saturated fats, found in butter, bacon, beef, whole milk, almost any food of animal origin and in coconut and palm oil, raise LDL levels. But polyunsaturated fat of vegetable origin of the omega-6 fatty acid variety, especially corn, safflower, soybean and sesame oils, tends to lower the LDL levels.

One of the best sources of polyunsaturated fats is in fish, especially cold water fish like salmon, trout, mackerel and cod. Researchers are discovering that fish oils actually lower levels of cholesterol and other blood fats associated with heart disease. The type of polyunsaturated fatty acids predominant in fish oil, omega-3, is two to five times more potent in lowering blood cholesterol than the omega-6 fatty acid variety. Omega-3 fatty acids may also make blood thinner, slower to clot and less likely to contribute to atherosclerosis. Studies show that omega-3 fatty acids may also lower blood pressure, ease common skin disorders such as eczema and psoriasis, relieve arthritis and aid brain development.

Besides diet, another cholesterol link is stress. Studies have shown that the cholesterol levels of medical students peak at exam time, while accountants hit their highest cholesterol levels around April 15 of each year, the deadline for filing income taxes in the United States.

Gender is another factor. Males and

females start out with the same cholesterol levels, but around puberty, boys experience a 20 to 25 percent drop in the protective HDL's and a threatening rise in LDL's. In some people, extremely high cholesterol levels are caused by a genetic defect. People with this condition, familial hypercholesterolemia, or others with less extreme tendencies to high blood cholesterol, are deficient in structures called LDL receptors, which sit on the surface of cells and remove the potentially harmful LDL cholesterol from circulation.

High blood *triglycerides*, also a lipid (fatty) material in the body, are an important risk factor. Some doctors think that the ideal triglyceride level is 100 mg. average 100-150 mg. and elevated above 150 mg. Since eating can elevate triglyceride levels, a 14-hour fast before having triglyceride levels tested should be observed.

In summary, there are several risk factors which are scientifically known to contribute to the development of coronary artery disease. Most of these can be controlled, at one level or another, to at least delay the consequences of the disease.

A Natural Cleansing Process For Arteries

One of the most interesting facts that has been discovered in recent years through scientific research has been an illumination of the process by which arteries become narrowed and finally clogged up with deposits including cholesterol. Even more importantly, we now understand how the body may clean its own arteries naturally.

Medical Research and Cholesterol

Several years ago, medical researchers became aware of the relationship between high blood levels of cholesterol and coronary artery disease. As more and more evidence began to accumulate against cholesterol, there was debate a few years ago over the benefits of reducing dietary cholesterol, since cholesterol can be made by the body from other substances. Later, the weight of medical opinion focused on both dietary cholesterol and high levels of blood cholesterol as being major risk factors.

Then, a few pioneering medical researchers discovered that cholesterol and other fats are carried in different forms in the bloodstream by other molecules: Low-density lipoproteins (LDL's) and high-density lipoproteins (HDL's). Researchers realized that the ratio of high-density lipoproteins to low-density lipoproteins or to total blood cholesterol was one excellent predictor of whether or not someone would develop coronary artery disease. People who had high levels of HDL's relative to the LDL's or total cholesterol had less chance of developing coronary artery disease.

HDL's help remove cholesterol from the body's cells and the lining of the arteries and carry it away to the liver for storage or removal. LDL's contain more cholesterol than HDL's. These molecules are less soluble in the blood and, therefore, their cholesterol can be readily deposited in the inner linings of arteries. Michael S. Brown and Joseph L. Goldstein received a Nobel prize in 1985 for their work showing how LDL receptors, like those in the liver, work to remove cholesterol from the blood and transform LDL molecules into HDL molecules or promote the formation of HDL molecules.

Recent studies indicate that when the percentage of HDL's can be increased, the progress of coronary artery disease can be slowed down or arrested in many cases. Early efforts to increase HDL's may help prevent coronary artery disease. Most studies indicate that low saturated fat diets can help prevent the development of coronary artery disease, but don't clean out arteries which are already obstructed. However, a few researchers maintain that a very restricted program of diet, exercise and lifestyle changes can sometimes reduce atherosclerotic plaque over a long period of time.

Natural Cleansing of Arteries

The latest research, some of which is not considered to be "proven" at this point, indicates that the percentage of HDL's, and the natural cleansing of the arteries, may be increased by the following:

Not smoking.

Regular aerobic exercise — such as brisk walking, bicycling, swimming or running.

Moderate consumption of beer or wine — (moderate may be arbitrarily assumed to be no more than one drink per day) but only in people who get very little aerobic exercise. (The moderate consumption of alcoholic beverages does not seem to raise HDL levels in regular, long-distance runners.)

However, raising HDL levels by consuming alcohol may backfire. Taking alcoholic beverages, even in moderation, is <u>not</u> usually recommended by most physicians, because it increases other risk factors like body weight, glucose intolerance, blood pressure, accidents and potential for alcoholism.

Reducing the amount of saturated fat in the diet — such as the fat found in meat and dairy products.

Reducing the amount of total fat in the diet — including fried foods, salad oils, dressings, margarines, mayonnaise, nuts and "fatty" vegetables, such as olives and avocados.

Weight loss — in people who are overweight.

Increasing the amount of polyunsaturated fat — especially fish oil, in the fat which does remain in the diet. The Omega-3 polyunsaturated fats found in fish oil seem to be more effective in increasing the percentage of HDL's than the polyunsaturated fats which are found in vegetable oils which are more of the Omega-6 variety.

Eating foods which are high in dietary fiber — like whole grain products.

Dr. James Anderson, M.D., who is professor of medicine and clinical nutrition of the University of Kentucky Medical College advocates oat bran as being excellent for lowering LDL cholesterol as quoted in a *Saturday Evening Post* article:
"Water-soluble fibers, such as oats, seem in practice to be especially effective in lowering cholesterol . . .
"We went ahead and demonstrated that oat bran did lower cholesterol even more than our usual high-fiber diet. Our usual high-carbohydrate high-fiber diet lowers cholesterol by an average of 25 percent, which is not too bad, but *with oat bran we found we obtained about a 35 percent reduction in the serum cholesterol.* The exciting thing — although it needs further documentation — is that in our preliminary studies we observed that oat bran selectively lowered the bad guys, the LDL, while raising the good guys, the HDL cholesterol. You see, in the artery, the LDL cholesterol spews cholesterol into the artery for

plaque formation whereas the HDL cholesterol (the good guys) serves a scavenger function in picking up cholesterol.

"As a starter, we said 100 grams of oat bran a day. We haven't titrated downward, but maybe for people who don't have bad cholesterol problems, eating 25 grams of oat bran or 50 grams of whole oats a day would have favorable effects in lowering cholesterol."

These are a few suggestions that seem to be valid steps in halting the degenerative process of coronary artery disease. Discuss them with your doctor. If you are currently under a physician's care, be sure to consult him before making any changes in your current treatment or dietary program.

Standard Medical Advice To Prevent Coronary Artery Disease

Most medical authorities recommend the following natural methods for reducing the chances of developing coronary artery or heart disease:

Not Smoking

Smoking is one of the *controllable* risk factors in heart disease. Research indicates that heart attacks among smokers are three times greater than among non-smokers and *five* times greater for those who smoke two or more packs a day. The good news is that people who quit smoking, unless they already have an irreversible smoking-related disease, soon regain most of their vitality and life expectancy. The risk of heart attack for people who quit smoking is about the same as it is for non-smokers.

People who are most successful at giving up smoking are usually the ones who stop "cold turkey". Since nicotine is a drug, a longtime smoker who quits abruptly will suffer withdrawal symptoms. These include nervousness, irritability, mouth watering, a bad taste in the mouth, and the feeling that something necessary is missing. There are organized programs that may help.

If you agree with Mark Twain that, "It's easy to quit smoking; I've done it hundreds of times!" — here are a few methods that may help in quitting. First, if you aren't ready to quit now, be considerate of others. Remember, at one time smoking was considered a sophisticated, adult thing to do, but now it is generally socially unacceptable. Being near a smoker can be almost as harmful as smoking itself, and it is irritating to be around somebody else's smoke. So, make a point of not smoking when you're around someone who doesn't or at a business meeting or restaurant. Second, try not to inhale. It won't be easy at first, but the more you try, the easier it will be. Third, using a restrictive cigarette holder will cut down on the amount of tar and nicotine that goes into your system and will lessen the withdrawal symptoms. Fourth, prepare yourself for quitting altogether. Make a list including why you smoke and why you should quit. Also list what triggers your smoking. Last, set a date to quit. Look at the lists often, and you can begin to break the smoking patterns.

Other plans to break the cigarette habit include hypnotism, group therapy in which people trying to quit help each other, non-prescription drugs, and a prescription drug, Nicorcttc® chcwing gum. Nicorcttc® is especially helpful because it neutralizes the lift from nicotine. Addiction to nicotine is the biggest stumbling block to quitting smoking.

Avoiding cigarette smoke is the most important thing to do to prevent coronary artery disease and many other health problems. Even longtime smokers can add years to their life expectancy by giving up smoking.

Engaging In Moderate Physical Activity

Since the heart is a muscle, it should not be allowed to become soft and flabby. Some people view exercise as boring, but it doesn't have to be. You can exercise to music or an exercise tape, in a class, with a friend, or read while on a stationary bicycle. You can pass the world by as you walk or jog. You can swim laps in a pool or play tennis with friends. Many people can walk to work, climb stairs instead of taking elevators, or cut the grass by pushing a lawnmower instead of riding one.

There are many benefits from a positive exercise program. Besides reducing the risk of heart disease, it can lengthen your life. Studies confirm the fact that physical exercise as a lifetime habit contributes to a longer life. Exercise can also make you more energetic and increase your stamina. If you're not used to exercise, you may feel tired after a workout, but the real thing that wears us down is *stress*, and exercise relieves stress by relaxing the muscles that have become tense. Exercise makes the heart pump harder, forcing oxygen carrying blood through the arteries and veins. You also take in more oxygen by breathing faster, which results in more pep. After a while, the body gets used to exercise and performs better as you get stronger. Exercise will make you feel and look better. As you lose fat, your muscles become firm and your posture improves. Self-confidence develops when you have high energy levels and a better mental outlook; many people even report being able to think more clearly.

When beginning an exercise program, warm-up with slow, gentle stretches for at least five minutes. Cool-down the last five or 10 minutes by gradually slowing the intensity of your exercise. Be sure to wear the right type of shoes for the kind of exercise you select. The wrong shoes could result in shin splints or other problems in the ankles, back or knees.

Brisk walking is the type of exercise recommended by most doctors. It puts a moderate amount of stress on the heart and lungs and strengthens them instead of overstressing them.

The American Medical Association advises that any person planning exercise should have a medical examination by a physician before beginning the program. There are cautions to be taken, too. Besides the warm-up and cool-down periods, allow at least two hours after eating before exercise. Also, if the heart rate doesn't drop below 100 beats a minute 10 minutes after exercising, or if you have pains in the chest, jaw, or neck during exercise, or experience faintness, light-headedness, an irregular heartbeat, vomiting or nausea, see your doctor.

Losing Weight Gradually

If you are overweight, a moderate weight-loss program is important until normal weight levels are reached. Obesity is associated with increases in illness and death from coronary artery disease, diabetes, stroke, kidney and gallbladder disorders. It may also contribute directly to high blood pressure, which is a risk factor in heart disease and stroke. If you are overweight, it is because you consume more calories than you use. Whatever the reason for being overweight, you must help your body use more calories than you actually eat. By reducing calories by 500 a day you should lose about one pound per week if you maintain the same level of activity.

If you need to lose weight, you don't need to learn to diet; you need to learn how to eat. The most effective diet is one that meets all nutritional requirements, is easy to follow when away from home, curbs between meal hunger and leaves you with a sense of well-being. Your doctor is the best source of information for your specific diet needs, but here are some general guidelines: 1) plan your meals and eat only at designated times; 2) drink plenty of water; 3) chew each bite thoroughly; 4) don't skip meals; 5) trim fat from meat before cooking; 6) limit red meats, pork, whole milk products, breads, sugar, salt and grease; 7) steam vegetables or eat them raw; 8) avoid fried foods and processed foods; and 9) remember, your new eating lifestyle will result in your being healthier and happier.

An excellent program for losing weight and reducing dietary fat and cholesterol is "The Bran Diet". You can order a copy by sending $3.99 plus $2.00 shipping and handling to FC&A, 103 Clover Green, Peachtree City, Georgia 30269.

Reducing Blood Cholesterol Levels

It's a fact: reduction of blood cholesterol levels *will* reduce the rate of coronary heart disease. Researchers have observed that the levels of fats in the blood *can* be lowered by changes in the diet. Only extremely high cholesterol levels require drug therapy. Clinical tests indicate that each one-percent reduction in blood cholesterol levels nets a two-percent reduction in coronary heart disease rates. For example, a five-percent reduction in blood-cholesterol levels should reduce coronary heart disease rates by ten- percent.

The first step in lowering blood cholesterol levels is diet therapy and weight loss if you're overweight. A moderate exercise program may also be helpful. The dietary approach is to lower *total* fat, saturated fat and cholesterol consumption. Saturated fat, found in meats and dairy products, should be reduced to ten-percent or less of total calories, while unsaturated fats, such as fish and vegetable oils, may constitute as much as ten-percent of total calories. Not smoking may also help reduce total cholesterol levels.

Most authorities agree that all Americans, beginning at age two, should adopt a lower fat, lower cholesterol diet. Lifestyle changes may be difficult, but the motivation for a healthier life is encouraging.

Lowering High Blood Pressure

Even mild hypertension, left untreated, more than doubles a person's chance of a heart attack. Reducing high blood pressure through dietary means or, if necessary, treatment with drugs is standard medical advice. Reducing the amount of salt in the diet as well as the amount of fat, cholesterol and calories (in overweight people), not smoking and a moderate amount of exercise may help many individuals lower high blood pressure.

Anxiety, frustration and anger may also aggravate reactive hypertension. It's impossible to completely eliminate emotional strain, but it is possible to avoid some stressful situations.

Talking it out, working off your anger, taking time out for yourself, doing for others and learning to tackle one job at a time are only a few of the positive actions you can take to lower your emotional tension.

Again, these are suggestions that most medical authorities agree help to reduce coronary artery disease and its related problems. Discuss them with your own doctor to see which ones might relate to your current treatment program.

Unproven Risk Factors Which Some Researchers Claim May Cause Or Contribute To The Development Of Coronary Artery Disease Or Heart Attacks

The following risk factors are not as well documented by as many research studies as the ones listed previously. In medical science, the word "proven" usually means, first, that an experiment has been conducted in which an *experimental variable* has been compared to a *control,* and that the results of the experiment are considered to be *significant.* Then, if those results are confirmed by other researchers in other studies, the results are considered to be *proven* after a period of time has passed without new research "proving" it untrue.

As can be seen, it is difficult for medical researchers ethically to conduct studies involving human beings and disease in such a manner that the studies can be reproduced. It's easy to feed chickens a diet extremely high in cholesterol and to observe the fact that they will get artery disease, but the results of animal experiments can't be directly applied to human beings without the risk of error due to basic biological differences: a chicken is not a human. There are important medical experiments which can never be performed on human subjects; to do so would be unethical.

Therefore, studies which seek to determine the causes or factors causing heart and artery disease rely on such things as questionnaires, statistics, and inferences which may be made after looking at one group of people and comparing them to a different group of people. The results of such studies are often arguable. Results are not considered to be "proven" until many different studies all point to the same conclusion and when few, if any, studies seem to be contradictory. Even then, it may be years before most researchers and medical doctors completely accept a large body of evidence as positively identifying a risk factor for human disease.

In the years ahead, some of the following *unproven* risk factors may come to be accepted by the medical community and others may fall by the wayside. Some may remain uncertain because they aren't considered important enough for sufficient research to be done for them to be accepted or rejected.

Since the following factors are *possible*,

though unproven risk factors, we have decided to list them, even though they may not be fully accepted by the medical community at this time.

Drinking Water From Chlorinated Water Supplies

There is a theory that drinking water from chlorinated water supplies may be a risk factor leading to coronary artery disease. This idea is based upon the fact that chlorine is a gas which theoretically could damage the walls of the arteries or cause other damage to the body or to food before or after it is eaten, even in very small concentrations. Chlorine is a reactive gas like carbon monoxide; carbon monoxide is one component of cigarette smoke which may damage arteries.

The evidence for this theory is largely circumstantial. Studies indicate that Eskimos, whose diet is composed mainly of animal fats, but whose drinking water is pure melted snow or ice, are practically immune to heart disease. Also, every community around the world that is *free* of coronary artery disease drinks unchlorinated water.

In Roseto, Pennsylvania, the drinking

water used to be from flowing mountain springs, with no chlorine residual added. Before its water supply was merged with the chlorinated water of its neighboring town, Bangor, Pennsylvania, it was reported that these people of Italian descent (who tended to be obese and whose diet was abnormally high in animal fats) used to be immune to heart attacks.

In the 1960's, experiments were performed on 100 male chickens. The chickens were divided into two groups and given the same food. The control group was given pure distilled water to drink. The other, the experimental group, had a heavy dose of chlorination added to their drinking water. Within three weeks there were major effects in both appearance and behavior in the experimental chickens. Subsequent autopsies revealed atherosclerosis in the chickens who were given chlorinated water, but no arterial abnormalities in the control group.

The evidence for chlorination being a factor in causing atherosclerosis is largely circumstantial, but it should not be ignored.

Low-Fiber Diets

One hundred years ago, the diet of the American people contained an adequate amount of natural food fiber. Most bread was made with whole wheat flour which contained bran, the outer, fibrous part of the wheat kernel. Coronary heart disease was rare at this time, and few people were troubled with appendicitis, diverticulosis, cancer of the large bowel, constipation, hemorrhoids or obesity.

Then, in the last quarter of the 19th century, American industry made two portentous discoveries which were hailed as breakthroughs in the march of progress. The first invention was the development of high-speed steel roller mills for flour milling. Food companies could then produce a fine white flour which tasted better than most whole wheat flour and which was less subject to spoilage. The second development was the growth of the canning industry; this processing greatly reduced food fiber content.

These two changes took place over a period of several years, and no one noticed that anything was wrong. But then, in the 20th century, scientists became puzzled at the persistent rise in certain death rates and obesity in the American people. Commentators noticed that people in backward countries didn't suffer very much from these ills.

In the 1940's and 1950's, a British surgeon, Dr. Denis Burkitt and other medical doctors like Cleave, Trowell and Heaton, noticed in East Africa that they never found a case of diverticular disease or cancer of the colon in thousands of rural tribesmen whom they autopsied. They checked further and found that obesity, appendicitis, heart attacks, constipation and hemorrhoids were also extremely rare. They thought that the amount of fiber in their diet prevented these ailments; so they investigated what happened to fellow tribesmen who moved to African cities or Britain and adopted a typical, low-fiber western diet. The results confirmed their hypothesis. On a diet that had been depleted of bran and other fiber, many Africans became obese and developed all the other ills of western man.

Here is what Dr. Denis Burkitt had to say on the subject of fiber and coronary artery disease in an address given in 1984 to an audience of physicians. More of this speech is quoted in *The Fiber Man* by Denis Burkitt and

Brian Kellock.

"Coronary heart disease kills one man in four in Britain. We did not see one case a year in our teaching hospital in Uganda ...

"Here is a quote from the standard medical textbook of 1920, the ninth edition of Ostler's Principles and Practice of Medicine: 'Angina pectoris (angina for short) is a rare disease in hospitals. One case a year is about average, even in the large metropolitan hospitals in London'.

"One patient a year! And yet today there are those who deal with this problem, so obviously due to modern Western culture, by giving people new hearts or plastic hearts. It is hard to think of anything more brilliantly irrelevant to the problem ...

"Protein intake in Britain and America has hardly altered in the past 100 years, the period over which these diseases have emerged. So I'll not spend time on proteins.

"As people get Westernized they always reduce their carbohydrate intake. Nearly half the carbohydrate intake in Britain now is sugar. There has been a catastrophic drop in starch, whereas the third world gets nearly 80 per cent of its energy this way. If you want to live a long and healthy life, get far more of your energy from starch: bread, flour products, cereals, beans and peas and root vegetables, particularly potatoes.

"Reduced starch intake is always accompanied by an increase in fat. We eat three times more fat than communities with a minimum prevalence of the diseases I have listed. We must reduce our fat. If I were a benevolent Czar and I could make a few edicts, one of them would be to abolish french fries. If you don't like your neighbor, then give him your frying pan! ...

"The biggest nutritional catastrophe in this country in the past 100 years had been the deliberate removal of fibre. We did not understand its nature or properties and had no way of measuring them. We thought it was cellulose. We gave it to the cattle. Third-world countries eat 60-140 grams of fibre a day. We usually eat under 20 grams. As a result our stool output has dwindled. We have a laxative industry in this country only because we have taken the fibre out of our food. We have got to get it back.

"We have also drastically reduced our grain consumption. In England we are nearly at the bottom of the European bread-eating league, eating about a quarter of a pound of bread a day each. Our ancestors ate about a pound and a half. Until very recently only 10 per cent of our bread was brown or wholemeal. Things are getting better. In Holland it is now over 50 per cent. In Denmark it is over 70 per cent.

"So eat more bread. If I could advise one change in your diet to improve your health it would be to eat two to three times as much bread. Not white. But brown or wholemeal.

"What does fibre do to your gut and mine? I can only touch on it briefly tonight. If you put fibre into a glass of water, what happens? It absorbs water and swells. In the gut fibre will hold the water partly by mechanical attraction and partly by providing food for the bacteria which are 89 per cent water anyway. So fibre ensures the presence of a large soft, easy-moving mass. It is strongly protective against constipation, and by this and other means provides protection against many diseases of the gut."

Here are quotes from a letter which Kenneth Heaton, M.D., wrote to The American Journal of Clinical Nutrition in February, 1976.

"Overnutrition is the factor which most firmly links a fiber-depleted or refined diet with raised blood lipids and heart disease.

"There is much and increasing evidence

that coronary heart disease (CHD) is essentially the result of habitual overnutrition.

"Overnutrition is usually equated with *too much* eating, and is blamed on self-indulgence. Yet to most people, overeating is surely an unpleasant experience and is followed by a compensatory period of abstinence. In spite of this, most civilized people habitually ingest more calories than they need or want. The paradox is resolved if this overnutrition is blamed on *too easy* eating, that is, on a diet which evokes a physiological level of satiety but only after an unphysiological excess of calories has been ingested. Overnutrition would then be a disorder not of people but of their diet.

"The manufacture of nearly all of our familiar carbohydrate foods (sugar, white, flour, corn and rice breakfast cereals, etc.) involves the removal of tough, fibrous material. This results in products which are physically easier to eat, because they need less chewing, than their unrefined or whole counterparts. No chewing at all is required with fiber-depleted sugars, which can be drunk. Because they need less chewing and lack non-nutritious bulk, refined foods are also less satisfying for a given energy intake and to many people they are more palatable. For these reasons (argued more fully elsewhere (5), fiber may be regarded as a natural obstacle to, or brake on, energy intake. Foods depleted of fiber must be regarded as intrinsically fattening because they are inadequately satisfying; any person who relies on them to satisfy his appetite inevitably ingests excess calories . . .

"There are strong grounds, therefore, for regarding CHD [coronary heart disease] as a disease caused largely by eating fiber-depleted foods. Sucrose must be singled out for special blame as it is the most refined, and so most easy to eat, of foods. It is also compulsively attractive to many people, and this is widely exploited in modern food and drink technology."

As can be seen, low-fiber diets are associated with higher risk of coronary artery disease in numerous studies. However, low-fiber diets are also associated with high-fat diets. Therefore, it is difficult to say if the *addition* of fiber to the diet without *reducing* the amount of fat and sugar in the diet would promote lower rates of coronary artery disease. Many researchers who are familiar with the latest studies feel that the absence of dietary fiber, particularly mushy types of fiber such as that found in oat bran, is a contributing factor which leads to the development of coronary artery disease.

Here are some high-fiber recipes from "The Bran Diet", a manual published by FC&A.

How To Prepare Brown Rice

1) Wash the rice by pouring cold water over two cups of brown rice until dust rises to the surface of the water. Pour off water, and repeat if necessary.

2) Add 3 cups of water to the clean rice and bring to a boil fast.

3) Cover pot and boil slowly for 45 minutes or until all water is absorbed.

4) Turn off heat and let steam for 10 minutes.

5) Keep the rice in the refrigerator and reheat it at mealtime.

Cod And Rice Bake

Combine 1 lb. of chopped cod, 3 stalks sliced celery, 1 chopped onion, 2 cups of stewed tomatoes, 1 cup of uncooked brown rice, 1-1/2 cups of mushroom soup.

Preheat oven to 325 degrees and bake for 1

hour and 20 minutes in a covered teflon casserole dish. Use 1-1/2 cups per serving.

Oatmeal And Raisins

Bring 1 cup of water to a boil. Add 3/4 cup of "old fashioned" not "quick" or "instant" rolled oats. Continue to boil for 1 minute then turn off heat and let simmer for 4 more minutes. Sprinkle a few raisins over oatmeal and serve.

Cereal And Fruit

Select a whole grain cereal that has little or no sugar or fat added to it. (Read the list of ingredients on the label.) Serve 2 oz. of cereal with 1 cup of skim milk, and add sliced fruit such as strawberries.

Homemade Bran Bread
(and Dinner Rolls)

9 cups of stone ground whole wheat flour
1 cup of unprocessed bran
2 packages of yeast
1/2 cup honey
2 egg whites
2-1/2 cups of skimmed milk

1/2 cup water
1/2 teaspoon salt

Let yeast stand in lukewarm, but not hot, water for 5 minutes. Boil milk and then add honey. After 5 minutes of cooling, put into mixing bowl with 2 egg whites, yeast and two cups of flour. Stir or beat, and add 1 cup of bran. Add rest of flour and salt gradually as you knead the dough. If dough is still sticky, knead in more flour. Place dough in a bowl and let rise uncovered for 1 hour and 45 minutes; then put in 2 non-stick loaf pans or roll pans. Let rise again for 1 hour. Bake loaves for about 40 minutes at 350 degrees. Bake rolls for 10 minutes at 425 degrees.

Bran Muffins

2 cups whole wheat flour
1-1/2 cups pure unprocessed bran (*note)
2 tablespoons honey
1-1/4 teaspoons baking soda (omit if flour is self-rising
2-1/4 cups buttermilk
1 egg white
1/2 cup dark molasses

Combine flour, bran, honey and soda. Mix well. Combine remaining ingredients and stir into dry ingredients, just enough to moisten. Spoon into non-stick muffin tins filling them 2/3 full. Bake at 350 degrees for 20 to 25 minutes. Makes 2 dozen muffins.

(*Note: Pure, unprocessed bran is different from 100% bran cereal. You can use either type in the recipes, but the products will have a slightly different texture.)

High-Protein Diets

Some researchers claim that the breakdown products of methionine (an amino acid found in protein) can damage the walls of arteries unless sufficient vitamin B6 is present. Since vitamin B6, which is found in meat, is partially destroyed by the cooking of meat, there is a theoretical basis for the idea that high-protein diets could be a risk factor even if such diets were not also high in fat. Like low-fiber diets, diets which are high in protein are also linked to diets which are high in fat, and high-fat diets are a known risk factor. Therefore, it is difficult to prove that excessive protein in and of itself is a risk factor for coronary artery disease.

Being Underweight

Some studies show that excessively thin people have higher rates of coronary artery disease and higher death rates than people who are close to normal weight. It is possible that higher death rates among thin people may be partially or completely related to smoking, a known risk factor which influences weight loss.

Altitude

Another possible risk factor is the altitude at which one lives. A study was conducted in New Mexico, where the altitude varies between 2,800 and 3,600 feet above sea level. It was found that the higher the altitude, the lower the death rate from heart disease. A possible explanation is that activities at higher altitudes require increased physical exercise.

"Type A" Personality

People who have hard driving, impatient "Type A" personalities may have an increased risk of coronary artery disease than those with easygoing, "Type B" personalities, but some studies question if such a relationship exists.

Type A people are very time conscious, always doing two jobs at once, often appearing to be in a self-induced race. They seem to go through life as quickly as possible, fearing they will miss something if they sit back and relax. Type B personalities, on the other hand, can be as productive as type A's, but type B's have fewer heart attacks, tend to talk slower, smoke less and have lower cholesterol levels.

On the other hand there is also some evidence that type A's seem more likely to survive heart attacks than type B's. The reasons the risk of heart disease may be higher for type A's may be that their blood has a strong tendency to clot under stress, that they stay under stress much of the time, or that they are more likely to smoke or overeat.

Homogenized Milk

The enzyme, xanthine oxidase, is found in high concentrations in the butterfat of milk (and also in lower concentrations in other foods). There is a theory that xanthine oxidase damages the arteries and contributes to coronary artery disease.

During the homogenization process, the

large particles (or globules) of fat naturally found in whole milk are broken down into many small globules. These small particles then stay disbursed throughout the "skim" portion of the milk, and no longer rise to the top of the milk as "cream".

Xanthine oxidase may be absorbed more readily from the small fat globules found in homogenized milk than in the large fat globules which are found in milk which has not been homogenized. Homogenization is now a standard procedure in the dairy industry, and it is difficult to find milk which has not been homogenized.

Because excessive consumption of saturated fat, which is found in high concentrations in milk and most milk products, has been positively identified as a risk factor in coronary artery disease, it may be difficult to determine how much damage xanthine oxidase does to the arteries and how much damage is caused by excessive butterfat. Research is continuing in this area.

Herpes Infections

Researchers have noted that people who

have a history of recurrent fever blisters or cold sores may be at extra risk for coronary artery disease. This leads to the theory that herpes infections, which linger in the body throughout the lifetime, as well as other viral infections may damage the arteries during outbreaks.

Dietary Mineral Imbalances

Geographical areas where the concentration of the trace element *selenium* in the water supply is low have high rates of coronary artery disease, heart attacks and cancer. Areas which are low in *chromium* also have higher rates of heart attacks. *Potassium* deficiencies may contribute to heart attacks. Areas which are high in *sodium* or *cadmium* have higher rates of heart attacks. But in areas where the drinking water is hard (higher concentrations of minerals like *magnesium* and *calcium*), there is less incidence of heart attacks. These patterns of disease, which are developed from geographical population studies, suggest that certain minerals may help prevent heart attacks and that other minerals may increase the risk of heart attacks.

Some findings indicate that *magnesium* deficiency is an important factor in congestive heart disease, heart attacks, angina, arrhythmia, strokes, high blood pressure, epilepsy and migraine headaches. *Magnesium* is one of the body's major electrolytes, along with *potassium, calcium* and *sodium,* and has been used in treating heart arrhythmias.

Caffeine

Caffeine is the substance that gives you that little boost in your morning coffee. Actually, that energy is nervous stimulation, because caffeine is a stimulant to the nervous system.

Caffeine may be a risk factor, because it can elevate blood fat levels, raise pulse rates and reduce tolerance for stress. Excessive caffeine can cause irregular heartbeats. People with heart disease, high blood pressure or especially unstable angina may be advised to avoid it. A recent study of patients having unstable angina showed higher heart attack rates in those who drank coffee than in those patients who didn't drink coffee. But for most people, caffeine in moderation (the equivalent of two or three cups of coffee per day) is not a proven risk factor.

In summary, only time will tell which of these factors are actually risk factors.

Unproven Methods For Treating Or Preventing Coronary Artery Disease

It takes time for promising new research studies to be confirmed, and even more time for the results to filter down to physicians who are treating patients. Therefore, the fact that a particular method of preventing or treating coronary artery disease is *unproven* does not mean that it is necessarily *unsound*. Some of these methods eventually may be proven to be effective, and others shown to be ineffective.

The unproven methods mentioned here (as well as any others that aren't discussed, such as eating raw onions or garlic to prevent blood clots) should be tried only with a doctor's advice. Use common sense, and check with your doctor. Don't neglect proven techniques of prevention like not smoking, lowering blood pressure and reducing cholesterol and saturated fats. Also, **do not** discontinue any medication unless directed to do so by your physician.

Relaxation Training

Relaxation training may help to lower blood pressure, reduce stress and lower the tendency of blood to clot in some people, especially the "Type A" personality. Avoiding stressful situations such as arguments, high pressure work or other tension-producing situations is helpful.

One study shows that listening may also take a load off the heart. Most people experience a rise in blood pressure when they speak, followed by a rapid drop when they listen. The study indicates that the louder and faster a person talks, the higher the blood pressure. Learning to listen may reduce stress.

<u>Taking Extra Vitamins</u>

Some researchers have suggested taking extra *niacin*, *folic acid*, *vitamin E*, *vitamin C*, or pyridoxine (*vitamin B-6*) to reduce levels of blood cholesterol or to protect against coronary artery disease. Many of the claimed benefits are based on studies where the vitamins were given in extremely high doses which can cause serious side effects. Vitamin B-6 and folic acid both may cause damage to the nervous system when given in high doses. Extremely high doses of vitamins C and E may cause higher death rates. High doses of niacin cause temporary flushing of the skin, itching, high blood sugar and other side effects.

Niacin given in high doses has been shown to reduce the amount of cholesterol in the blood. In a recent study of heart attack victims, it was found that those who took high doses of niacin had an 11 percent lower death rate than those who did not. Niacin must be administered in high doses to be effective against cholesterol and heart disease, but because of the significant side effects, it should be taken only under a doctor's supervision. Some people — those with diabetes, gout or ulcers — should not take niacin at all.

Research on vitamin E indicates that it may inhibit blood platelet clumping, by protecting the endothelial cells (cells that line the inside of the arteries). The protected endothelial cells can continue to produce a substance called prostacyclin, which discourages platelet aggregation, resulting in less chance of blood clotting.

Vitamin C may be helpful, too. It may also inhibit platelet clumping. These vitamins should also only be taken under a doctor's supervision. Large doses can be harmful.

Taking Extra Minerals

Taking extra *chromium, selenium* or *magnesium* has been suggested as a way of reducing coronary artery disease. This theory is based on studies which show that people who live in areas of the country where these minerals are low in the water and soil have higher rates of coronary artery disease and heart attacks than people who live in areas of the country where these minerals are in good supply. Since selenium can be quite poisonous in relatively small doses, most medical authorities recommend great caution in adding selenium to the diet.

Magnesium, considered to be relatively harmless when taken in levels close to the RDA, seems to regulate the balance of calcium and sodium in our cells, particularly in our heart and blood vessels. It is believed that magnesium deficiencies are a likely factor in many diseases or conditions that involve constriction or spasm of the heart and arteries system. An adequate intake of magnesium may help the heart to beat smoothly and regularly and withstand the stress of daily life, while also helping blood vessels remain open and relaxed, thus lowering blood pressure.

Any addition of minerals to the diet safely should be made only at the Recommended Daily Allowance (RDA) level. Ideally, one should adjust intake of vitamins and minerals by eating a wholesome diet and not by relying on supplements.

Aspirin

A recent study has confirmed that aspirin can reduce the chance of having a second heart attack in people who have already had heart attacks. Aspirin reduces the tendency of the blood to clot and the chance of clots forming. It has also been used successfully by physicians to treat unstable angina, a condition thought to result from the incipient clogging of an already damaged coronary artery.

Studies show that aspirin seems to help previous heart attack victims, but this doesn't mean that it's good for everyone. It remains to be seen if "an aspirin a day for all" will help people protect against heart attacks.

Drinking Chlorine-Free Water

Drinking chlorinated water is a possible, but unproven risk factor. Some researchers believe that chlorine is a cause of atherosclerosis. Some people recommend drinking pure hard water from a deep, health department inspected well or commercially available mineral spring hard water, if it can be positively ascertained that the water is certified "pure" from a source that is not subject to contamination. Mountain Valley Water from Hot Springs, Arkansas, has a good balance of beneficial minerals.

One way to remove chlorine is to boil tap water then let it cool; boiling drives off the chlorine, although it may leave behind chlorinated hydrocarbons. Activated charcoal filters, unless they are of the large, under-the-sink type, may not remove all of the chlorine or chlorine byproducts from tap water. Also, microorganisms may grow in the filters and possibly contaminate the water.

Eating Cold Water Fish

The oil found in some fresh water fish and all salt water fish, especially cold water fish like salmon, mackerel, cod and trout has been discovered to be beneficial in raising HDL levels. Population studies show that people who eat substantial amounts of cold water fish have lower rates of coronary artery disease than other people, even if the total amounts of fat in the diets of both groups is about the same. Recent studies suggest that the addition of fish to the diet and especially the replacement of much red meat and dairy products with fish would be a positive health benefit which may reduce the chance of developing coronary artery disease.

Fish oil supplements don't provide nearly as much fish oil as is obtained by eating fish, unless you gobble pill after pill. Fish oil supplements like cod liver oil can be harmful when taken in large doses because of the large doses of fat soluble A and D vitamins which they contain. Only caution about eating fish: watch out for bones!

Ultra-Low-Fat Diets

The American Heart Association recommends that the percentage of fat in the typical American diet be lowered from around 42 percent of calories to around 30 percent of calories. Many physicians and authorities think that it's better to lower the amount of fat in the diet, especially saturated fat, to drastically lower levels. These same people advocate diets which are moderate in protein, low in salt and high in dietary fiber. Such diets are composed mostly of vegetables, starchy, whole-grain complex carbohydrates, such as whole wheat breads and cereals, brown rice, potatoes, fish, plus some fresh fruit and very low amounts of low-fat dairy products and red meat.

There is much evidence that such diets really work, not only to prevent or retard the development of coronary artery disease but, in some cases, to retard further damage in people who already have it.

Many medical authorities are skeptical of claims that diet can reduce already existing artery plaque. Studies of people who go on diets, like vegetarian diets, where the amount of saturated fat has been greatly reduced, do not usually show any reduction in atherosclerotic plaque or in already existing coronary artery disease. Nevertheless, authorities do not yet agree as to whether a stricter diet and fitness program can sometimes reduce atherosclerotic plaque. Isolated cases of plaque reduction have been documented in some people who have gone on a program that includes: 1) not smoking; 2) gradual weight reduction and weight control in overweight people; 3) regular, aerobic exercise; and 4) an ultra-low saturated fat, moderate calorie, complex carbohydrate, low salt, high dietary fiber diet with small meals and healthy between meal snacks like apples or crisp vegetables.

Such a diet and exercise program was advocated by Nathan Pritikin, a nutritionist who died recently. Pritikin was said to have been diagnosed as having coronary heart disease, angina and high blood cholesterol levels 30 years before his death, but a confirmed diagnosis can't be documented because inadequate records were kept. After much research, he put himself on a radical program like the one described above. When he died, his body was autopsied. The attending physician was, in his own words, "amazed to find no evidence of coronary artery disease in a man of his age".

Many people with coronary artery disease, high blood pressure or diabetes who have attended the Pritikin Centers and gone on their medically supervised program of diet, exercise and appropriate weight loss have reported remarkable results. Some patients are able to be taken off medication. Many of them reportedly feel better and experience relief from angina. Because of the successes at the Pritikin Centers and similar successes elsewhere, the trend in the medical community is to re-evaluate the American Heart Association guidelines and to seriously consider the benefits of a stricter low fat, low salt, high complex carbohydrate diet plus regular aerobic exercise.

Please check with your physician before beginning any diet. Weight reduction diets are not recommended for pregnant women or people with certain diseases.

Modern Medical Treatment Of Heart And Artery Disease

Most doctors would prefer to treat coronary artery disease by preventing it through lifestyle changes. However, if artery disease already exists, drug treatment is usually prescribed. In advanced cases of artery disease, surgery may be used to maintain the life-giving flow of blood to the heart.

Treatment for heart disease is not always straightforward. There is currently much debate among physicians about when it is advisable to operate and when it is better to treat a patient with drugs. New studies are being released almost daily, and some of these studies are challenging some currently routine procedures. The medical treatments listed here are those treatments that doctors presently may use.

Testing

To determine if drug treatment, lifestyle changes or surgery will be advised, doctors use a variety of tests. These tests help locate blockages or partial blockages in the arteries and aid in determining how much stress the heart is experiencing. From these tests, the doctors have a better idea of the best way to treat existing coronary artery disease.

Exercise or Stress Test — The purpose of this test is to see how your heart and circulatory system work under physical stress. Most times, the patient's heart is monitored while running or walking on a treadmill or while riding a stationary bicycle. An EKG is often given during an exercise or stress test and compared to an EKG of the resting heart.

EKG — An electrocardiograph (EKG or ECG) is a recording of the heart's electrical activity. The usual short form for the electrocardiograph, EKG, comes from the Greek root word, kardia By placing electrodes, usually with gel, on a person's arms, legs and chest, the heart's electrical activity can be monitored. This activity is printed on a strip of graph paper. The EKG forms a long graph of up and down rhythms or waves of the heart. A normal heart produces a certain pattern. By studying the shape, size and time of the heart's impulses, it is often possible to locate and diagnose various heart rhythm problems. An EKG is often used to determine if a heart attack has occurred or is occurring.

If you have had serious heart trouble, you may want to keep a wallet sized card copy of your most recent EKG with you. If a medical emergency occurs, doctors can compare an emergency EKG to your wallet-sized one and make a more accurate diagnosis of your situation. Wallet-sized cards are available from EKG Alert, PO Box 2337, Quincy, MA 02269.

Holter Monitoring — This is actually a mobile, lightweight EKG machine. It is attached to a person to get 24-hour heart rate recording in his/her regular surroundings and activities. Heart rhythms are recorded on magnetic tape and matched against a diary that the person keeps. Some heart problems only occur occasionally, and the Holter monitor has made it easier to spot them.

Echocardiogram — An ultrasound picture of the heart, an echocardiogram, may be used to see artery blockages or discover physical abnormalities of the heart and valves. Like an EKG, the echocardiogram can record the heart's movement for further study. In this test procedure, nothing is attached to the body. The person lies quietly on a table, and ultrasound waves are passed through the body and bounced back to a small, hand-held receptor; since sound waves are "painless", the only thing the patient feels is the receptor smoothly rolling back and forth over the skin. The bounced-back sound waves, or echoes, are recorded to make a graphic picture of how the heart is working. This tells the doctors more about the way the heart functions and makes it easier to provide the best care and treatment.

Arteriogram — An arteriogram (or coronary angiograph) is a special x-ray picture of an artery after injection of a dye. This test is often used to determine if someone has suffered a heart attack, needs bypass surgery, or how well surgery recovery is progressing. A radiopaque dye, called a "contrast medium", is injected into a catheter which has been inserted into the artery in question. The dye allows the flow of blood in the arteries to show up on x-rays so it can be examined. Obstructions in the heart, arteries or veins will be seen by the doctors.

A catheter is a long, thin, very flexible tube which can be moved through the inside of arteries or veins. In a special procedure called cardiac catheterization, the catheter is inserted into a large artery in the thigh and carefully maneuvered up to the heart. When the dye is injected into the catheter, it flows to the heart, and a picture of the heart valves, chambers and vessels is visible by x-ray.

Injecting x-ray dyes by heart catheterization can cause dangerous side effects like blood vessel spasms, irregular heart rhythms, heart attacks, blood clots, allergic reactions or strokes. It is a procedure which should be used sparingly.

Venogram — An x-ray of the veins, taken after a contrast dye has been injected and is flowing in the veins, is similar to an arteriogram.

Electrophysiological Testing — Programmed Electrical Stimulation (PES) is sometimes used to determine which drug would be most effective in an individual with an irregular heartbeat. In the test, the doctor electrically stimulates the heart into an irregular pattern. Then he uses one of the drugs being tested and records that drug's effect. The process is repeated with various drugs, if necessary, until the best drug for that patient is found.

Drug Treatment

Existing cases of coronary artery disease may be treated with a variety of drugs that a physician thinks are appropriate. These include blood pressure reducers, diuretics (water pills), heart rhythm regulators, and other drugs which can be helpful in alleviating conditions like angina pectoris. Modern drug treatments are proven to reduce the chances of having a heart attack, but they're not a cure-all, because they frequently produce undesirable side effects.

Drug treatment is quite complex because many people have more than one ailment and need several different drugs. The interaction of those drugs and the actions that the drugs have on the body have to be considered for each person, so drug treatment must be individualized. For example, some people with angina may also have high blood pressure, high levels of blood cholesterol or congestive heart failure.

Here are some brief descriptions of the major drug groups used to treat heart problems. We have included the drugs used to control high blood pressure, because high blood pressure causes undue strain on the heart and blood vessels, which contributes to heart problems. The drugs are listed with the generic (or chemical) name first, followed by the brand names. The most widely used drugs are listed in detail at the end of this chapter with their intended effects, side effects, warnings and interactions.

ACE Inhibitors — ACE is an abbreviation for *angiotensin converting enzyme inhibitor*. ACE inhibitors cause the ACE enzyme to "bind" in the body. When the ACE enzyme is not available, blood pressure is maintained at a regular level. When the blood pressure is maintained, the heart docsn't have to work as hard. This is a new class of drugs that has been just introduced in the 1980's.

- captopril (Capoten®)
- enalapril (Vasotec®)

Anticlotting Drugs (nicknamed "blood thinners") — These drugs reduce the ability of the blood to clot and help to protect people against fatal blood clots.

- anisindione (Miradon®)
- dicumarol (Dicumarol®)
- phenprocoumon (Liquamar®)

121

- warfarin potassium (Athrombin-K®)
- warfarin sodium (Coumadin®, Panwarfin®)

Blood Fat Reducers (technically called "antilipidemics") — These medications serve to lower the levels of cholesterol and triglycerides in the blood, which helps to prevent or slow down the effects of hardening of the arteries.

- cholestyramine (Questran®)
- clofibrate (Atromid-S®)
- colestipol HCl(Colestid®)
- dextrothyroxine sodium (Choloxin®)
- gemfibrozil (Lopid®)
- nicotinic acid (Vitamin B3/Niacin — various brands available)
- probucol (Lorelco®)

Blood Vessel Enlargers (medically termed "vasodilators") — These chemicals act on the small arteries of the body, causing them to relax. This reduces their resistance to blood flow, and blood pressure goes down.

- cyclandelate (Cyclospasmol®, Cyclan®)
- ethaverine HCl (Ethaquin®, Ethatab®, Ethavex-100®, Isovex®, Circubid®)

- isoxsuprine HCl (Vasodilan®, Voxsuprine®)
- nicotinyl alcohol (Roniacol®, Rontinol®)
- nylidrin HCl ((Adrin®, Arlidin®)
- papaverine HCl (Cerespan®, Pavabid®, Pavatym®)

Beta Blockers — *Beta-adrenergic blocking agents* affect the heart muscle by blocking the action of naturally occurring substances, like norepinephrine and epinephrine, that stimulate the heart. These substances, which are released into the circulation in response to physical exertion or other stress, cause an increase in heart rate and in the force with which the heart pumps blood. This, in turn, causes an increase in oxygen demand. By decreasing the rate and force of heart contraction, beta blockers reduce the heart's workload and therefore reduce its oxygen demand. Beta blockers are often used in combination with nitrates for the long-term treatment of people with stable angina.

- acebutolol (Sectral®)
- atenolol (Tenormin®)
- metoprolol (Lopressor®)
- nadolol (Corgard®)

- oxprenolol (Trasicor®)
- pindolol (Visken®)
- propranolol (Inderal®, Inderal® LA)
- timolol (Blocadren®)

Blood Pressure Reducers (medically termed antihypertensives) — These drugs act in a variety of different ways to help lower high blood pressure levels.

- clonidine (Catapres®)
- guanabenz (Wytensin®)
- guanadrel (Hylorel®)
- guanethidine (Ismelin Sulfate®)
- hydralazine (Apresazide®, Ser-Ap-Es®, Unipres®)
- labetalol (Normodyne®, Trandate®)
- methyldopa (Aldomet®)
- metoprolol and hydrochlorothiazide (Lopressor HCT®)
- minoxidil (Loniten®)
- prazosin (Minipress®)
- reserpine (DemiRegroton®, Duipres®, Hydromox R®, Regroton®, Serpasil®, Unipres®)
- rescinnamine (Moderil®)

Calcium Channel Blockers — These medicines interfere with the transport of calcium into the heart and vein muscle cells and inhibit their contraction. This causes the veins and arteries to enlarge and reduces heart rate.

- diltiazem (Cardizem®)
- nifedipine (Procardia®)
- verapamil (Calan®, Isoptin®)

Diuretics (often called "water pills") — These are chemicals which act on the kidneys, causing them to flush salt and water from the body. As fluid volume in the blood vessels drops, the blood pressure also goes down.

- amiloride (Midamor®)
- bendroflumethiazide (Naturetin®)
- benzthiazide (Exna®, Hydrex®,)
- bumetanide (Bumex®)
- chlorothiazide (Diuril®)
- chlorthalidone (Hygroton®,
    Thalitone®)
- cyclothiazide (Anhydron®, Fluidil®)
- ethacrynic acid (Edecrin®)
- furosemide (Lasix®)
- hydrochlorothiazide (Esidrix®,
    HydroDIURIL®)
- hydroflumethiazide (Diucardin®,
    Saluron®)
- indapamide (Lozol®)

- methyclothiazide
  (Enduron®, Aquatensen®)
- metolazone (Diulo, Zaroxolyn®)
- polythiazide (Renese®)
- quinethazone (Hydromox®)
- spironolactone (Aldactone®,
  Aldactone®)
- trichlormethiazide (Metahydrin®,
  Naqua®)
- triamterene (Dyrenium®)
  combinations - Moduretic®,
  Spironazide®, Dyazide®

Heart-Rhythm Regulators (medically termed antiarrhythmics) — These drugs slow and strengthen the heartbeat and correct irregular heart rhythms.

- amiodarone HCl (Cordarone®)
- digitalis glycoside (Crystodigin®)
- digoxin (Digoxin®, Lanoxin®,
  Lanoxicaps®)
- disopyramide (Norpace®, Norpace
  CR®)
- flecainide acetate (Tambocor®)
- mexiletine HCl (Mexitil®)
- phenytoin (Dilantin®)
- procainamide HCl (Procan®,
  Pronestryl®)

- quinidine gluconate (Quinaglute®)
- quinidine polygalacturonate
  (Cardioquin®)
- tocainide (Tonocard®)

Nitrates — These chemicals produce vasodilation (widening of the blood vessels) mainly of the veins but also of the arteries. Nitrates are part of the blood-vessel enlargers drug group and have been a main form of angina therapy for more than 100 years. The main effect of nitrates, however, is to reduce heart muscle (myocardial) oxygen demand. When the veins farther away from the heart (peripheral veins) are dilated, less blood reaches the heart's chambers; this reduces cardiac workload and therefore reduces the heart's need for oxygen.

The most common blood vessel enlarger is nitroglycerin. Since nitroglycerin is often needed very quickly, it is available in several different forms: in an ointment that is rubbed on the chest, in patches with the ointment already measured and attached, in sublingual tablets that are placed under the tongue to dissolve, in an aerosol spray that is sprayed in the mouth, in chewable tablets, in tablets that are swallowed, or in oral tablets that will slowly release the nitroglycerin into the body. A topical drug is one that is placed on the outside of the body, like an ointment or cream. A systemic drug is one that is swallowed and released into the whole body's system.

- erythrityl tetranitrate (Cardilate®)
- isosorbide (Isordil®, Sorbitrate®)
- nitroglycerin - systemic (Nitrostat®, Nitro-Bid®, Nitrolingual®)
- nitroglycerin - topical (Nitrol®, Nitro-Dur®, Transderm-Nitro®)
- pentaerythritol tetranitrate (Peritrate®, Peritrate® SA)

Potassium Supplements — Potassium is a mineral that is sometimes needed to offset the side effects of some blood-pressure reducing drugs, which lower the body's potassium to below normal levels.

- Kay Ciel®, K-Lor®, K-Lyte®, and Micro-K Extencaps®

Chelation Drugs — WARNING: Non-Prescription Chelation Therapy For Circulation Problems Is Illegal — The "chelation" (pronounced ke'la'shen) products that are being sold door-to-door, through the mail, and over-the-counter are not true "chelation" therapy, according to the FDA. They are various mixtures of vitamins, minerals and amino acids that have no proven benefit for treating or preventing heart, artery or circulation (cardiovascular) problems.

Advertisers say these drugs will reduce arterial plaque or hardening of the arteries, explains Arthur Auer, an FDA Compliance Officer. However, Auer warns that these oral drugs are NOT an alternative to bypass surgery, doctor prescribed medications, or drugs that are injected directly into the arteries.

"The oral products may be safe but they are not effective against vascular disease," Auer warns. The FDA has not approved a non-prescription oral chelation product. They are now classified as "unapproved new drugs" and their sale must stop, he said.

True chelation therapy is controversial and not recommended by most doctors for treating hardening of the arteries. This therapy uses agents that combine with or "bind" to metals in the body. They are used to combat poisonings with heavy metals, digitalis overdoses and excess calcium, the FDA explains. With this therapy, doctors inject the FDA approved chelating drugs directly into the bloodstream.

The FDA is advising people to stop taking any home use "chelation" therapy.

Surgical Treatment

Heart Bypass Surgery — In certain people, coronary artery bypass surgery may be the best treatment. This technique, which was first used in the late 1960's has become increasingly popular and now is considered an almost routine procedure in many hospitals.

Despite its popularity (*Business Week* magazine reports that some 125,000 bypass operations were performed in a recent year), this surgery is definitely not for everyone. Surgery is a serious trauma to the body and should only be considered if the problem cannot be controlled by lifestyle changes or drug treatment. The latest recommendation is that the operation is of value when there is a severe narrowing in more than one coronary artery or where the left main coronary artery is severely obstructed. If a person is operated on by a physician who has had good success in bringing his or her patients through the operation and recovery period, the recovered patient may experience relief from angina and also a slightly improved life expectancy. Ideally, the surgeon should be a physician with a good reputation who works at a major medical center, where hundreds of bypass operations are performed each year.

In heart bypass surgery, the doctor takes a large vein from one of the legs (usually the saphenous vein) and uses it to go around a clogged coronary artery supplying the heart muscle. The leg vein is attached above and below the clogged portion of the artery. The blood will then flow through the "bypass" and avoid the clogged area. By diverting the blood, the heart is relieved from oxygen starvation, and the pain of angina should decrease. Sometimes, the bypass is achieved by using a mammary artery from the chest.

Doctors often refer to the number of bypasses that will be performed during surgery as single, double, triple, quadruple or multiple bypass surgery. The numbers explain how many bypass shunts will be used.

Unfortunately, some patients don't survive the operation. Other patients who do survive the operation sometimes have problems with the bypasses tending to clog up over the months or years ahead. Usually within ten years, the replacement vein will become blocked, just like the artery that originally caused the problem. Even if the surgery goes well, a recent report, the *Coronary Artery Surgery Study*, says that bypass surgery doesn't necessarily prolong life.

New studies indicate that the internal mammary arteries, which go down the side of the rib cage just behind the breastbone, may be better than leg veins for grafting during bypass surgery (*New England Journal of Medicine*, January 2, 1986). The studies indicate that since mammary arteries do not clog up as quickly as the leg veins, they may last indefinitely. Researchers in the study found that people who had a bypass operation with a vein had a 60% higher risk of death, over a ten year period, than people who had bypass surgery with an artery graft. Because of placement problems, mammary artery grafts aren't always feasible.

Other Bypass Surgery — Arteries farther away from the heart, especially those in the legs, may become blocked and require bypass surgery. Bypass surgery away from the heart is called a "peripheral" bypass. Rather than using an artery or vein from another part of the body, most peripheral bypasses use artificial arteries made of Dacron®.

Angioplasty (also called balloon angioplasty or percutaneous transluminal coronary angioplasty) — A balloon-tipped catheter is inserted into an artery, usually in the leg. The catheter is carefully pushed and guided to the obstructed area of the coronary artery. The balloon is then expanded to a predetermined size and contracted several times, which helps to crush the plaque and widen the blood vessel. With the widened blood vessel, proper blood flow can be restored in the artery. Angioplasty is effective 90% of the time, but it's only used on 10% of bypass candidates to reduce the rate of possible complications. With good physicians, angioplasty has a much lower fatality rate than bypass surgery. It's also faster, far less expensive and requires only a short recovery period.

Unfortunately, there is no guarantee that the block or obstruction will not recur. Angioplasty may need to be repeated more often than bypass surgery. Even though angioplasty has far less risk and expense than coronary bypass surgery, it is usually recommended for patients who only need a single bypass and not for those who need a double, triple or quadruple bypass. Angioplasty is most successful on the left anterior descending coronary artery and on people who have had angina only for a short time. An experienced team, like Dr. Jay Holman's team at the Cleveland Clinic, is desirable for successful angioplasty. Dr. Holman studied under the late Dr. Gruntzig, the pioneer of coronary angioplasty.

Researchers are now working on new angioplasty techniques that involve laser or scalpel excision of atherosclerotic lesions. Researchers hope these new techniques will provide a better way to open the blocked passage and keep it open.

Valve Replacement or Repair Surgery — Replacing or repairing any of the valves of the heart requires opening the heart and is considered to be very major surgery.

Vein Stripping — Vein stripping is removing or tying off the aggravated, damaged veins. Healthy veins usually take over for the veins that are tied off. Vein stripping is done in a hospital under general anesthesia. Elastic bandages will then need to be worn for several days. Stripping of varicose veins is now considered to be of questionable value in many cases, and other treatments are often used.

Implanting An Artificial Pacemaker — Over 100,000 patients in the U.S. receive heart pacemaker implants each year. If an irregular heartbeat is related to problems of the sinus (or sinoatrial) node, which controls the pace of a healthy heart, an implanted pacemaker is usually the best treatment.

Pacemaker electrodes are usually implanted within the heart itself. Its tiny generator is implanted under the skin in the upper chest. Before the recent advances in technological miniaturization, the pacemaker was not implanted but worn externally. A pacemaker emits an electrical impluse, like a healthy sinus node does, which stimulates the heart to beat an average of 72 beats per minute.

The newest pacemakers use lithium batteries which keep working for about ten years. Each pacemaker's pulse rate and time between beats is individually set for the person who will be using the pacemaker. Now, some pacemakers can be changed and controlled from outside the body.

Implanting An Electric Defibrillator — The implanted defibrillator can stop potentially fatal disturbances in the heart's rhythm by delivering a jolt of electricity to the heart when its rhythm becomes irregular. This is a relatively new device that was approved by the FDA in the fall of 1985 with the hope that it could possibly prevent between 10,000 to 20,000 deaths per year in the United States. The defibrillator is different from a pacemaker. The pacemaker works constantly to get a slow heart rate up to a normal level, while the defibrillator only reacts in sudden and acute situations.

The defibrillator's electrical pulse generator is larger than a pacemaker and is about the size of a deck of cards. Several electrical leads connect the generator with the heart muscle. Within the pulse generator are microcircuits that sense the intrinsic rhythm of the heart. When an irregular heartbeat begins, the pulse generator sends a series of electrial impulses to the heart to reestablish the normal rhythm. The defibrillator's actions can be monitored by radio, by the person's doctor, so he can tell how the device is functioning and how many times it has had to shock the heart muscle. The person may have had no idea that the defibrillator has been active.

Presently, the battery in an implanted defibrillator only works for two years, and then must be replaced by surgery. But researchers hope that the length of the battery life will be increased and that the size of the defibrillators will be decreased in the future.

Checklist Before Surgery

If your doctor recommends that you need surgery, here are several things to remember:

1) Time is very important, but so are the risks you will be facing if you have the surgery. Get a second opinion, from an impartial heart doctor, before you proceed with surgery. Heart surgery involves great risks, and you should be sure that these risks are necessary. Many insurance companies are now requiring a second opinion for major surgery.

If you are unsure about how to get a second opinion, you can call the Second Surgical

Option Hotline run by the Health Care Financing Administration at (800) 638-6833 or (800) 492-6603 in Maryland. They will give you names of local doctors who have agreed to act as a second opinion consultant. These doctors will not profit by your surgery and should be an impartial judge of whether or not the surgery is necessary.

2) Once you have been assured that surgery is necessary, choose your doctor carefully. Doctors who work at major hospital centers, where hundreds of similar operations a year are performed, may have much lower fatality rates than other doctors. Check into your doctor's record with other patients having surgery similar to yours. Try to talk to other people your doctor has treated. Did the doctor communicate well before and after surgery? Did the patient understand all the procedures? Make sure that you feel comfortable with your physician and that you can talk to him/her. Check his reputation with other doctors. Ask him what his fatality rate is.

3) Prepare yourself to be an excellent patient. Learn all you can about the surgery. Ask your doctor very specific questions, prior to surgery. . . How long will you be in surgery?

Will you stay in an intensive care unit (ICU) or coronary care unit (CCU) after the surgery? How long will the recuperation period be after surgery? Plan to leave your job in capable hands, so that you can relax and recuperate. You won't need the extra stress of your work if you want to recover properly.

Don't be afraid to ask financial questions ahead of time. If you have insurance, get at least twenty claim forms before surgery. Get the insurance person at the doctor's office to outline the kind of charges that will be expected. Ask questions. Where will the charges be coming from? Who will bill for the diagnostic tests, the anesthesia, the hospital stay, the physical therapy after surgery, the doctor's fees? What does my insurance cover? How long do I have to pay for the procedures my insurance doesn't cover?

4) Before you go to the hospital, make arrangements to have someone speak for you if you are not conscious. This may be your spouse, a close relative or friend. This is just a precaution, but if something unusual happened during surgery and you couldn't speak for yourself, decisions will need to be made. Ask your doctor (and perhaps your lawyer) about

the best way to arrange for this.

5) Take your doctor's office and home phone numbers with you to the hospital and make sure your next of kin have them too. You will need to feel assured that you can get in touch with your doctor whenever you need to.

6) After surgery, eat and exercise as recommended by your doctor. It is foolish to pay thousands of dollars and risk your life with surgery, then turn around and ignore your doctor's recuperation plan.

This chapter has described many of the standard tests and treatments. Next, we will examine some treatment alternatives which are being tested and developed.

Treatment Options For Coronary Diseases: Current And Experimental

Treatment Alternatives For Specific Problems

This chapter focuses on a number of the most common and serious aspects of heart disease. Standard medical treatment options are described, as well as some of the most recent, ongoing research and experimental approaches.

Angina Pectoris

1. Drugs — to widen the arteries (nitroglycerin and nitrates); to decrease the heart's workload (calcium channel blockers and beta blockers); to decrease the formation of blood clots and break up existing clots (aspirin and "blood-thinners").

2. Newest Drug Treatment — Aspirin inhibits the action of small cell fragments in the blood called platelets, which have a role in blood clotting. In this way, aspirin is thought to decrease the likelihood of a heart attack. In patients with unstable angina, an aspirin a day reduced the risk of getting a heart attack, or of dying of a heart attack, by about half (from a

12% chance without aspirin to a 6% chance with aspirin), in a recent three-month study reported by the Food and Drug Administration.

Nitroglycerin, a blood-vessel enlarger, is now available in an aerosol spray. The new aerosol version is available by prescription as Nitrolingual® (by Rorer). It is sprayed, in a regulated amount, directly onto the tongue where it is quickly absorbed into the blood stream. Researchers hope that the spray will provide quicker, longer-lasting relief than the current, widely-used tablets.

3. Surgical Treatment — bedrest, bypass surgery or angioplasty.

Atherosclerotic Peripheral Vascular Disease

1. Drugs — to decrease the formation of blood clots and break up existing clots (anticlotting drugs, commonly called "blood-thinners").

2. Surgical Treatment — bypass surgery, where the blocked artery (most often in the leg) is replaced with an artificial artery

Atherosclerosis (hardening of the arteries)

1. Drugs — to widen or dilate the arteries (nitroglycerin and nitrates); to decrease the heart's workload (calcium channel blockers and beta blockers); to decrease the formation of blood clots and break up existing clots (anticlotting drugs).

2. Surgical Treatment — angioplasty or bypass surgery.

Blood Clots

1. Drugs — to decrease the formation of blood clots and break up existing clots (anticlotting drugs).

2. Surgical Treatment — angioplasty or bypass surgery.

Congestive Heart Failure

1. Drugs — to help slow heartbeat and make heartbeat stronger (heart rhythm regulators); to help remove excess fluid from the body and reduce the strain on the heart (diuretics).

2. Surgical Treatment — surgery to repair aneurysms, to implant a pacemaker, or to repair or replace heart valve.

Heart Attack (Myocardial Infarction)

1. Emergency Medical Treatment — quick medical treatment is essential. CPR and electrical defibrillation may be needed. Patient will be given oxygen and plenty of rest to stabilize the emergency condition. An EKG will be used to monitor and determine the damage caused by the heart attack. Blood tests may be necessary, including testing the activity in the white blood cells to see if the immune system is working to clear away the cells that have been damaged during the heart attack.

2. Drugs — to reduce pain (pain relievers); to calm the patient and relieve anxiety (sedatives); to decrease the formation of blood clots (anticlotting drugs); to help slow heartbeat and make heartbeat stronger (heart-rhythm regulators); to maintain regular heartbeats (heart-rhythm regulators); to help remove excess fluid from the body and reduce the strain on the heart (diuretics); to widen the arteries (nitroglycerin and nitrates); to decrease the heart's workload (calcium channel

blockers and beta blockers).

3. Newest Drug Treatment — An aspirin a day reduces the chance of having another heart attack, or of dying from another heart attack, by about one-fifth, according to new studies released by the FDA. A daily aspirin is only recommended for people who have had a heart attack, not as prevention against a first attack.

Inderal® (propranolol) may "lengthen the lives" of many heart attack victims by reducing the chances of a recurring heart attack during the early recovery period. This is a new use of the beta-blocker drug Inderal® based on a three-year study by the National Heart, Lung and Blood Institute. The manufacturer of Inderal®, Ayerst Laboratories, introduced it in 1967 for the treatment of irregular heartbeats. Since then Inderal® has been approved for treatment of high blood pressure, angina, and migraine headaches.

Streptokinase, t-PA, and APSAC are experimental drugs used immediately after a heart attack to dissolve life-threatening clots.

4. Surgical Treatment — bypass surgery may be necessary.

High Blood Pressure (Hypertension)

1. Drugs — to help remove excess fluid from the body and reduce the strain on the heart (diuretics); open or dilate the blood vessels (nitroglycerin and nitrates); to decrease the heart's workload (calcium channel blockers and beta blockers); to reduce the blood pressure levels by various ways (blood pressure reducers); also mineral supplements (potassium) are often necessary to reduce the effects of the thiazide diuretics and combinations of all these drugs.

2. Newest Drug Treatments — Vasotec® is a new ACE (Angiotensin Converting Enzyme) inhibitor that may be taken only once-a-day. Researchers hope that the one-a-day doses, combined with fewer side effects, will make Vasotec® a great addition to available blood pressure reducing drugs. Its chemical name is enalapril maleate/MSD (manufactured and developed by Merck Sharp & Dohme).

Trasicor® (oxprenolol HCl) is a new beta blocker. Like other beta blockers, Trasicor® has the ability to control a variety of heart-related disorders. In recent studies of high blood pressure patients, Trasicor® effectively lowered blood pressure when taken only once daily. Further studies show that Trasicor® produces a lower incidence of some side effects, especially wheezing, than other beta blockers.

One particular drug, labetalol HCl (Normodyne® by Schering, and Trandate® by Glaxo) combines in a single medicine, the beneficial properties of two main classes of drugs, beta blockers and blood vessel enlargers, which are now used to control high blood pressure. Taking the best from each class, labetalol HCl:1) lowers blood pressure quickly without excessive increase in heart rate and 2) helps stabilize the heart rate and blood pressure during stress or exercise.

Lopressor HCT®, by Geigy Pharmaceuticals, is a new drug combination of the widely used blood-pressure reducer Lopressor® (metoprolol) and the diuretic hydrochlorothiazide (the generic drug also sold as Esidrix® and HydroDIURIL®). This new formulation means that many people taking two different drugs will now have to take only one tablet.

Drug treatment for mild to moderate high blood pressure has been extremely controversial within the medical profession. Doctors do not agree at what level the blood pressure must be to start drug treatment.

But in a new study that Dr. Charles Hennekens presented to an American Heart Association meeting in San Francisco, early drug treatments are shown to save lives. People with mild high blood pressure who took drugs had 40% fewer fatal strokes and 38% fewer non-fatal strokes. Therefore, treating mild or moderate high blood pressure with drugs may save lives.

3. Surgical Treatment - no surgical treatment is required unless the high blood pressure creates other diseases.

Irregular Heartbeats (Arrhythmias)

1. Drugs — to maintain regular heartbeats (heart-rhythm regulators); to decrease the heart's workload and eliminate extra heartbeats which originate in the heart's lower chambers (beta blockers).

2. Newest Drug Treatment — Mexiletine (Mexitil® by Boehringer Ingelheim) has been approved as a new heart-rhythm regulator.

Mexiletine is chemically similar in structure and action to lidocaine, the intravenous medication used in hospitals for irregular heartbeat. It works well in combination with other drugs because it can be used in lower doses that do not cause unwanted side effects.

Tonocard® (tocainide) by Merck Sharp & Dohme is an oral drug which works the same way as lidocaine. Until the introduction of Tonocard®, patients suffering from major heart problems, such as heart attacks, congestive heart failure, hardening of the arteries and narrowing of the heart valves, had to return to a doctor or hospital when their heartbeat became very irregular. With Tonocard®, many of these people can be treated on an outpatient basis.

Tambocor® is another new heart-rhythm regulator. It is an alternative to Tonocard® which is also used to decrease chances of heart failure in heart attack survivors. Researchers at Riker, who developed Tambocor®, claim it is more effective and has less side effects than Tonocard®. Tambocor® is also the first heart-rhythm regulator to be given in just twice daily doses.

Amiodarone HCl (Cordarone® by Wyeth)

is a "a drug of last resort" for patients who are "at great risk". This drug should only be used by experts in treating heart rhythm disorders "after attempts to use alternative agents have failed", according to the FDA.

3. Surgical Treatment — if the irregular heartbeat is related to the sinus node (a particular portion of the heart muscle where the heartbeat originates), surgery to implant a pacemaker may be required. In some cases of serious heartbeat irregularities that don't respond to drug treatment, an electric defibrillator may be implanted.

Rheumatic Heart Disease

1. Drugs — using penicillin at the first sign of strep throat before the actual outbreak of rheumatic fever (which is an allergic reaction strep-caused disease) helps to prevent heart damage.

2. Surgical Treatment — in extreme cases, surgery to replace heart valves.

Strokes

1. Emergency Medical Treatment — support breathing, reduce blood pressure levels, stabilize fluid levels in the body, and provide rest.

2. Drugs — to help remove excess fluid from the body and reduce the strain on the heart (diuretics); open or dilate the blood vessels (nitroglycerin and nitrates); to decrease the heart's workload (calcium channel blockers and beta blockers); to decrease the formation of blood clots and break up existing clots (anticlotting drugs).

3. Surgical Treatment — to prevent strokes, removal of blockages from carotid arteries (the neck arteries that take the blood to the brain).

Thrombophlebitis (Blood Clot With Inflammation Of The Vein)

1. Drugs — to decrease the formation of blood clots and break up existing clots (anticlotting drugs); to reduce pain (pain relievers); to reduce inflammation and swelling (anti-inflammatory drugs).

2. Surgical Treatment — usually drugs and bed rest with the clotted areas elevated are enough to prevent trouble. However, if drugs cannot be used on some people, angioplasty or actual removal of the clot may be necessary.

Varicose Veins

1. Drugs — to decrease the formation of blood clots and break up existing clots (anticlotting drugs); to reduce pain (pain relievers).

2. Surgical Treatment — if the varicose veins stop the blood supply to the legs or cause great pain or discomfort, surgery (called vein stripping) may be used.

A chemical is now being used to close off veins as an alternate to vein stripping. The treatment, known as a sclerosing solution, is injected into the vein and causes that vein to close. It takes four to six weeks after surgery for the vein to completely compress. This chemical injection method has more complications than vein stripping, and so it is not as popular. If the veins become a problem again, surgery is recommended, rather than another chemical injection.

New Treatment Possibilities Now In Research

Lasers — Using lasers to destroy blockages in the arteries is now in the experimental stage. A laser is attached to the end of a catheter, and then using a small TV picture, the doctor uses the laser to dissolve the fat and plaque.

However, it is very difficult to direct the laser beam to the exact spot, because veins and arteries don't conform to straight lines like the laser beam. If the laser beam misses the clogged place, it can hit an arterial wall and cause serious damage.

A new technique for laser treatment is being tested by doctors at Boston University Medical Center. Instead of having the laser beam hit the blockage, the beam is used to heat a small metallic probe shaped like an inverted V (similar to an arrowhead). The heated probe is then used to vaporize the blockage. As a small path is made in the artery, balloon angioplasty could then be used to break down more of the plaque.

LVAD (Left Ventricular Assist Device) — This is a heart pump that is similar to parts of artificial hearts. It is used to help strengthen hearts that are weak. Rather than replacing the natural heart, the LVAD works at the same time as the heart. Most LVAD's that are currently available are very large, about the size of an air conditioner, but researchers hope to develop a small LVAD that could be implanted, like a pacemaker, in a person with a weak heart.

Magnetic Resonance Imaging (MRI) — Magnetic resonance imaging is a new way of testing for and determining heart, vein and artery problems. MRI uses magnetic forces to view through the body and gives a three-dimensional picture of our internal organs. Because MRI uses our bodies just as they are, no special dyes or x-ray material needs to be injected into the veins, the imaging is safe and easy to perform.

Although there are relatively few centers that can now provide MRI because of the great initial investment required (about $1.5 million per MRI scanner), more will probably be available in the near future. Currently, pictures of the heart are blurry because of the heart's constant beating motion, but with research, MRI could become a great asset in evaluating heart disease.

Blood Tests For Heart Disease — New

blood tests that will warn us about high blood pressure risks and atherosclerosis may be available soon. These tests will detect if we are in a high-risk category for these diseases and start us on the road to prevention.

New, Experimental Drug Treatments

Mevinolin® is a new drug now being tested to raise the HDL and lower the LDL cholesterol levels. In clinical trials, blood cholesterol has been reduced by an average of 42% and triglycerides by 15%. These results are incredible, considering that according to *Cardiac Alert* newsletter, current diet and drug therapy usually drops the cholesterol levels only by 10%. Mevinolin® works by removing cholesterol from the blood and stopping the liver from producing more. It is still in clinical testing, but it is definitely a drug to watch for in the future.

Streptokinase — Streptokinase has the ability to activate the natural clot-dissolving properties in our blood system. In new treatment for heart attacks, streptokinase is inserted in a catheter, directly to the heart, where it works to dissolve the blood clots. It has been used in research for about 20 years, but it may not be the most effective new drug available.

t-PA is a new clot dissolving drug that could save lives of heart attack victims. According to a study at the National Institutes of Health (NIH), published in the *New England Journal of Medicine*, (312: 932-36) it has saved several lives and stopped permanent damage to many heart attack victims.

t-PA (tissue-type plasminogen activator) is made with new "genetic engineering" technology. It seems to have several advantages over presently approved drugs.

According to the published NIH study, t-PA is twice as effective as Streptase® (streptokinase) in opening up closed arteries of heart attack patients. The study involved nearly 300 people -- half took t-PA and half took streptokinase. In 1 1/2 hours, about two-thirds of the people who took t-PA had complete or partial reopening of their arteries, compared to only one-third of the streptokinase patients.

Another advantage is that t-PA can be injected into the veins. The majority of currently available clot-dissolving drugs must be injected directly into the heart arteries for maximum effectiveness. This technique, known as heart catheterization, requires very complex equipment and highly trained staff to perform the procedure.

Therefore, heart catheterization is very expensive and not available at every hospital.

Also, dissolving clots with streptokinase can release harmful substances, which can complicate recovery, in the area of the heart attack. Many heart attacks are caused by blood clots. Dissolving the clots could make the difference between a "minor" heart attack and major heart damage.

t-PA is still in the experimental stages, but if tests go well, it could be submitted to the FDA and approved within two or three years.

APSAC is a new drug that may be able to interrupt heart attacks soon after they begin, claims Beecham Laboratories, the drug's developer.

Up to 30% of heart attack survivors undergo such extensive heart muscle destruction during the first attack, that they suffer a second, fatal attack within a year, according to Beecham.

APSAC, like t-PA, is one of several drugs now being tested to help dissolve blood clots either during or immediately after a heart attack. It works by dissolving the sudden heart clots or "thrombi" that choke off the flow of oxygen to the heart. APSAC is technically known as Anisoylated Plasminogen Streptokinase Activator Complex.

Beecham says APSAC is different from other clot-dissolving drugs in use and under investigation, because it is long-acting and able to be given in a single 5-minute injection into a vein.

Some clot-dissolving drugs, like streptokinase and urokinase, must be injected directly into the heart (heart catheterization). According to Beecham, other drugs in the research stage, like t-PA, must be administered over several hours to be most effective.

Clinical trials of APSAC have begun in a number of major U.S. medical centers. To date, it has been tested in more than 600 patients worldwide.

Milrinone is a new heart-rhythm regulator that is being tested for use in people with congestive heart failure. It is similar to Inocor® (amrinone lactate).

Estrogen Replacement Therapy may be used for women past menopause to lower the rate of heart attacks. Estrogen is a hormone found naturally in a woman's body, but its levels fluctuate during different phases of a woman's life, declining drastically after menopause, and replacement therapy is sometimes required. According to *Cardiac Alert*, "four times as many postmenopausal women die from coronary artery disease as from breast and uterine cancer combined".

In summary, many of the drugs and techniques presented in this chapter are still being researched. Discuss them with your doctor if you have any questions as to how they might relate to your treatment program.

A Total Program For Preventing Coronary Artery Disease

A few years ago, the United States Government sponsored a $115,000,000 program called the Multiple Risk Factor Intervention Trial Study. In this program, several thousand people were enrolled and guided through several steps to lower the known risk factors for coronary artery disease. They ate less saturated fat. They took drugs to lower blood pressure, and they were counseled to give up smoking. The net health gain from this trial was exactly *nothing*. There was hardly any change in the mortality statistics (death rates) for people who were attempting to lower their risk factors. In fairness, it should be pointed out that a number of physicians have stated that, except for a higher than expected mortality among people who took diuretic drugs (water pills), the study as a whole did show a reduction in mortality.

Whether or not the study did or did not show a significant reduction in the death rate is beside the point. Even if it did show such a reduction, the reduction was relatively small compared with the overall problem of high death rates from artery disease and related

161

diseases of the circulatory system. Other attempts to lower risk factors have also met with limited success unless a *total* approach to the problem — a total change in lifestyle — is implemented. The only truly significant successes in reducing symptoms and death rates from coronary artery disease and other diseases of the circulatory system have been accomplished by the Pritikin Centers and other similar programs, where people enrolled are shown how to completely change their diet, exercise and lifestyle patterns. Even so, such programs, as good as they are, may not be able to mimic exactly the conditions which are best for preventing this illness.

Common sense would seem to dictate that any program to totally prevent degenerative artery disease should closely parallel the factors which are present in communities where artery disease is virtually non-existent. These are the primitive populations mentioned in earlier sections of this book. In these communities, the foods that people eat usually are complex, whole grain carbohydrates (starches) with lots of dietary fiber, little cholesterol or fat, and moderate amounts of protein. Whole grain products, as well as beans, peas, yams, sweet potatoes and other vegetables supply most of the calories and nutritional needs of these people.

Any red meat or dairy products which are eaten are a relatively small percentage of the diet, 10% or less. Fish, especially cold water fish, is a good source of animal protein, with other animal protein being provided from lean cuts of meat which are not overcooked. Infants and toddlers are fed as much as possible with mother's milk. Vegetables and fruits are eaten fresh, retaining all the natural vitamins and other nutrients. Calorie consumption is moderate and only enough to maintain a healthy, trim physique.

Drink is unchlorinated water, often from sources which are high in beneficial minerals like magnesium and calcium and low in harmful minerals. Exercise is daily, regular and of the aerobic variety. Smoking cigarettes and a host of dietary and drinking indiscretions are not problems.

There may be certain disadvantages' to the above lifestyle factors present in many primitive societies. One disadvantage (?) is that children in primitive cultures are generally short in stature, as were our ancestors in earlier centuries. Additionally, many nutritionists would question whether the diets of primitive peoples provide adequate nutrients, although other nutritionists who have studied nutrition in primitive communities might disagree. Thirdly, primitive people often suffer from waterborne parasites and bacterial diseases. Finally, primitive diets which keep blood cholesterol at low levels may increase the chances of cancer and possibly other diseases.

A total, medically supervised program for preventing coronary artery disease, which is similar to lifestyle factors present in primitive societies, could increase death rates from other causes. Nevertheless, lowering rates of coronary artery disease, or perhaps preventing almost all coronary artery disease, is so great a benefit that a possible, but as yet unproven, increase in death rates from other diseases is of small significance.

Any program to prevent artery disease by closely paralleling certain lifestyle factors in primitive cultures should be conducted under medical supervision as a controlled experiment because of the uncertainties.

Final Note

We hope that this book has shown you how coronary heart disease and other atherosclerotic diseases are avoidable for many people. We trust that you have discovered several measures you can easily take to reduce your risks. It makes sense to start a program of prevention as early as possible for this slowly developing disease.

If you have any questions about the information in this book, please talk them over with your physician. Self-treatment, especially in the case of a serious illness, is *not* a good idea. Even though natural methods of preventing atherosclerotic artery disease may be helpful, there is no substitute for management by a skilled physician if you already have artery disease or if you have ever had a heart attack.

The information provided in this book is based on the latest available *medical* testing, research and treatment, as well as other research reports of *natural* methods of prevention and treatment. But, we would encourage you not to overlook the *supernatural* power of God, from whom all healing comes. If you put your faith and trust in Him by believing in His Son, Jesus Christ, He will answer your prayers for healing according to His will. If you would like to know more about how to have eternal life through Jesus Christ, please write to:

FC&A
Dept. AGC 86
103 Clover Green
Peachtree City, Georgia 30269

Definitions And Explanations Of Terms Related To Heart And Artery Disease

Aneurysm — An abnormal weakness in the wall of a blood vessel, usually an artery. It is most often found in the aorta, which is the biggest artery in the body going from the heart through the chest and abdomen. An aneurysm can swell, enlarge, and eventually rupture.

Angina Pectoris — A sudden pain or pressure in the chest behind the breastbone which may radiate down the shoulder, neck, arm, hand, or back, usually or mainly on the left side of the body. People with angina pectoris may also feel its sensations as burning, choking, or like indigestion. It is associated with insufficient blood flowing through narrowed coronary arteries which supply the heart muscle.

Arrhythmia — An irregularity in the rhythm of the heartbeat.

Artery — Any blood vessel that carries blood away from the heart to the various organs and tissues of the body.

Atherosclerosis — The deposit of cholesterol

and other fatty, waxy substances on the inner walls of the arteries, often leading to narrowing and "hardening" of the arteries as scar tissue and calcification form.

Capillary — A minute blood vessel that connects the smallest arteries to the smallest veins.

Cardiac Arrest — Stopping of the heartbeat.

Cholesterol — A waxy fat present in some foods of animal origin; it is also manufactured by the human body. Some cholesterol is needed by the body, but excessive amounts are associated with artery disease.

Congenital Heart Disease — A malformation of the heart which is present at birth; a birth defect. Sometimes congenital heart defects can be corrected by specialized surgery.

Congestive Heart Failure — Occurs when the heart is unable to pump well enough to maintain good circulation, because of weakness of the heart muscle due to disease or a mechanical fault in the valves that control the flow of blood.

Coronary Heart Disease or Coronary Artery Disease — Narrowing or blockage of the coronary arteries which reduces the flow of blood to the heart muscle.

Coronary Insufficiency — Prolonged, insufficient blood supply to the coronary arteries; a condition having the symptoms of a heart attack, but without damage to the heart muscle.

Coronary Thrombosis — A blood clot in a coronary artery.

Heart Attack — Heart failure or abnormal, weak functioning of the heart after its blood supply is abruptly cut off, usually due to narrowing of the arteries or a blood clot.

Hypertension — Sustained high blood pressure of 140/90 or higher.

Myocardial Infarction — Death of heart muscle, usually in an area supplied by a coronary artery that is blocked. Also, sometimes used as a synonym for heart attack.

Rheumatic Heart Disease — Damage to the heart and especially the heart valves caused by rheumatic fever, which sometimes follows a streptococcal bacterial infection (such as an untreated strep throat) in which the body's immune response attacks the heart.

Stroke — An interruption of blood flow to an area of the brain, leading to damage and certain loss of function controlled by that area of the brain. Strokes can be caused by blockage of a blood vessel in the brain or by bleeding from a blood vessel or an aneurysm into the brain. The risk factors for stroke are similar to those for coronary artery disease. High blood pressure and smoking are leading risk factors for stroke.

Triglycerides — A type of fat carried throughout the body by the bloodstream; it is a particular combination of the 3 fatty acids, joined together. High trigylceride levels are associated with overeating, obesity, high-fat or high-sugar diets, diabetes and coronary artery disease. High levels are dangerous.

Vein — Any blood vessel that carries blood back to the heart from various parts of the body.

Bibliography

Anderson, James W., M.D. *Diabetes: A Practical New Guide to Healthy Living.* Arco Publishing, Inc., New York, NY. 1981.

Aviation Medical Bulletin. January, 1982 — December, 1985. Bill Maness, Editor. Harvey W. Watt, Atlanta, GA. 1985.

Bruhn, John G. and Wolf, Stewart. *The Roseto Story: An Anatomy of Health.* University of Oklahoma Press, Norman, OK. 1979.

Cawood, Gayle, M.Ed. et al. *Prescription Drugs' Side Effects Revealed.* FC&A, Peachtree City, GA. 1984.

Chilnick, Lawrence D. *The Pill Book of Heart Disease.* Bantam Books, New York, NY. 1985.

Ellis, Jeffrey W., M.D. and Editors of Consumer Guide®. *Medical Symptoms and Treatments.* Publications International, Skokie, IL. 1983.

Englebardt, Stanley L. *How To Avoid Your Heart Attack.* Reader's Digest Press, New York, NY. 1974.

Eyton, Audrey. *Fiber Man: The Life Story of Dr. Denis Burkitt.* Lion Publishing Corporation, Belleville, MI. 1985.

Gaby, Alan, M.D. *The Doctor's Guide to Vitamin B6.* Rodale Press, Emmaus, PA. 1984.

Hochman, Gloria. *Heart Bypass: What Every Patient Must Know.* Ballantine Books, New York, NY. 1982.

Kuntzleman, Charles T. *The Well Family Book.* Here's Life Publishers, Inc., San Bernardino, CA. 1985.

Likoff, William M.D., Bernard Segal, M.D. and Lawrence Galton. *Your Heart.* J.B. Lippincott, Philadelphia, PA. 1972.

Mayer, Jean. *A Diet For Living.* Pocket Books, New York, NY. 1975.

The Merck Manual of Diagnosis and Therapy. Merck
    Sharp & Dohme Research Laboratories, Rahway,
    N.J. 1982

Miller, Benjamin F., M.D. and Galton, Lawrence.
    Freedom from Heart Attacks. Simon & Schuster
    Inc., New York, NY. 1972.

Morrison, Lester, M.D., D.Sc., F.A.C.P. *Dr.
    Morrison's Heart-Saver Program.* St. Martin's
    Press, New York, NY. 1982.

Moskowitz, Mark, A. M.D. and Osband, Michael, E.
    M.D. *The Complete Book of Medical Tests.* W.W.
    Norton & Company Inc., New York, NY. 1984.

Price, Joseph, M.D. *Coronaries/Cholesterol/Chlorine.*
    Pyramid Books, New York, NY. 1971.

Pritikin, Nathan and McGrady, Patrick Jr. *The Pritikin
    Program for Diet & Exercise.* Grosset & Dunlap,
    New York, NY. 1979.

Pritikin, Nathan. *The Pritikin Promise: 28 Days to a
    Longer, Healthier Life.* Simon and Schuster Inc.,
    New York, NY. 1983.

Pritikin, Nathan. *The Pritikin: Permanent Weight-Loss
    Manual.* Grosset & Dunlap Publishers, New York,
    NY. 1981.

Seelig, Mildred S., M.D., M.P.H., F.A.C.N.
    *Magnesium Deficiency in the Pathogenesis of
    Disease.* Plenum Publishing Corporation, New
    York, NY. 1980.

Snider, Arthur J. *A Doctor Discusses Learning How to
    Live with Heart Trouble.* Budlong Press Company,
    Chicago, IL. 1982.

Watts, H. David. M.D. *Handbook of Medical
    Treatment.* Jones Medical Publications, Greenbrae,
    CA. 1983.